ATLAS OF
GASTROINTESTINAL
ENDOMICROSCOPY

ATLAS OF
GASTROINTESTINAL
ENDOMICROSCOPY

Yan-Qing Li

Shandong University, China

Khek-Yu Ho

National University Hospital, Singapore

Xiu-Li Zuo

Shandong University, China

Cheng-Jun Zhou

Shandong University, China

World Scientific

NEW JERSEY • LONDON • SINGAPORE • BEIJING • SHANGHAI • HONG KONG • TAIPEI • CHENNAI

Published by

World Scientific Publishing Co. Pte. Ltd.

5 Toh Tuck Link, Singapore 596224

USA office: 27 Warren Street, Suite 401-402, Hackensack, NJ 07601

UK office: 57 Shelton Street, Covent Garden, London WC2H 9HE

British Library Cataloguing-in-Publication Data
A catalogue record for this book is available from the British Library.

ISBN-13 978-981-4366-65-6
ISBN-10 981-4366-65-X

Typeset by Stallion Press
Email: enquiries@stallionpress.com

Printed in Singapore.

Contents

Prologue

The advent of confocal laser endomicroscopy in 2004 has had a major impact on the diagnostic algorithm of gastrointestinal endoscopy. Diagnosis in endoscopy is composed of three steps: recognition, characterization, and confirmation. First, recognition of subtle or flat mucosal changes is essential and high definition endoscopy helps identify these changes. Second, characterization of the mucosal pattern is necessary for predicting histology. The overall lesion type, vessel architecture, and surface pattern should be classified to predict histology, and several lesion and pattern classification systems are available for this purpose. Third, histology is needed to confirm the underlying disease and the rationale of endoscopic or surgical therapy. Historically, *ex vivo* histology of biopsy specimens was the gold standard for confirmation of a final diagnosis.

Endomicroscopy has revolutionized the final step of confirming a diagnosis and has broadened the diagnostic possibilities of gastrointestinal endoscopy toward functional and molecular imaging. It combines white-light imaging with confocal microscopy and provides subcellular resolution. It does not predict histology; it provides *in vivo* histology at subcellular resolution during the endoscopic procedure. It is a revolutionary technique which has significantly broadened the diagnostic spectrum of gastrointestinal endoscopy.

Endomicroscopy has helped us to better understand mucosal physiology and pathophysiology, leading to novel diagnostic algorithms based on newly discovered microscopic alterations of the gastrointestinal mucosa. Moreover, molecular imaging with antibodies and peptides has opened a completely new diagnostic field for gastrointestinal endoscopy. More research has to be done to fully cover the potential of endomicroscopy. However, a multitude of research activities all over the world have already clarified many diagnostically and clinically useful aspects of endomicroscopy.

Endomicroscopy is highly examiner-dependent and deep knowledge of histology and pathology is necessary in order to achieve competence. Formal endomicroscopic training by the key researchers will become vitally important for achieving expertise in endomicroscopy. The true value of endomicroscopy will emerge with the standardization of training and the *in vivo* classification of gastrointestinal diseases.

China and Singapore are major players in endomicroscopic research and practice, and play an important role in the continued development of the field of *in vivo* imaging. This English Atlas of Endomicroscopy, edited by Yan-Qing Li, Khek-Yu Ho, Xiu-Li Zuo, and Cheng-Jun Zhou (all internationally renowned experts in this field), is truly a milestone toward achieving proper training and teaching of endomicroscopy. It comprehensively reviews and summarizes all available research and clinical aspects, as well as the prospects of endomicroscopy. High quality endomicroscopy images can be viewed side by side with conventional histology, providing a great educational opportunity.

I am impressed with the outstanding quality of the *Atlas of Gastrointestinal Endomicroscopy*. This volume will give you an excellent opportunity to enhance your knowledge in the exciting field of endomicroscopy.

Ralf Kiesslich
Professor of Medicine
University of Mainz, Germany
May 2011

List of Contributors

Chuan-Lian Chu, MD

Xiao-Meng Gu, MD

Lim Lee Guan, MD

Khek-Yu Ho, MD

Rui Ji, MD

Yu-Lei Jia, MD

Chang-Qing Li, MD

Wen-Bo Li, MD

Yan-Qing Li, MD

Zhen Li, MD

Jun Liu, MD

Xue-Feng Lu, MD

Peng Wang, MD

Tao Yu, MD

Cheng-Jun Zhou, MD

Xiu-Li Zuo, MD

This book is funded by a key Clinical Project from the Health Ministry of China and the Taishan Scholar Program from Shandong Province of China.

Part 1

HISTORY

Chapter 1

The Development of Confocal Laser Endomicroscopy

Confocal laser endomicroscopy (CLE) is a newly introduced endoscopic tool that makes it possible to carry out confocal microscopic examination of the mucosal layer during ongoing endoscopy. The development of CLE is based on the technology of confocal laser microscopy.

In 1955, Professor Marvin Minsky invented the first set of confocal laser microscopes at Harvard University. Compared with the optical microscope, the confocal laser microscope has higher resolution, and can carry out a layering scan and 3D reconstruction of samples; the confocal laser microscope can also be used to observe the real-time dynamic state of live cells and obtain signals at the subcellular level. Therefore, the invention and application of the confocal laser microscope represented the beginning of a new era.[1]

In 1996, Professor S. Kudo predicted that the ability to establish an immediate endoscopic diagnosis virtually consistent with the histologic diagnosis would be the ultimate objective of endoscopists from the very early phases of the development of endoscopy. The high-resolution and live cell imaging techniques of confocal laser microscopy made the prediction possible.

In the late 1990s with the advent of miniaturization technology, the size of the confocal laser microscope was reduced (Fig. 1.1); later, it was further reduced so as to be integrated within the endoscopic lens body. Thus, the transition from confocal laser microscopy to confocal laser endomicroscopy was achieved.[2]

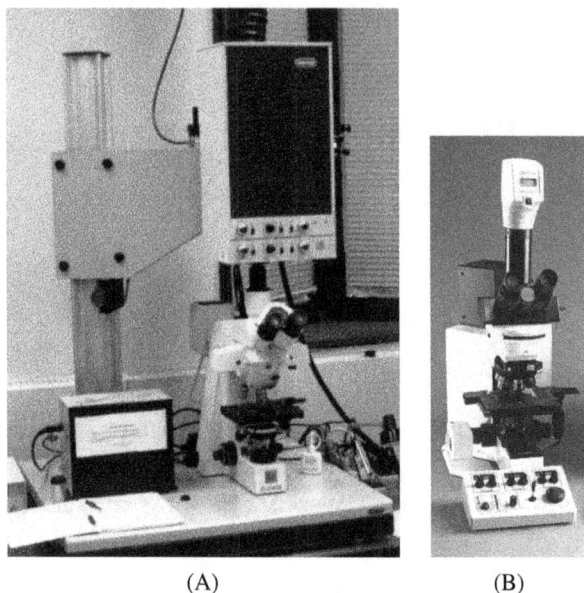

(A)   (B)

Fig. 1.1.   The evolution of the confocal laser microscopy volume. (A) BioRad MRC600 confocal laser microscope. (B) Optiscan optical fiber confocal laser microscope.

The initial confocal laser endomicroscope was rigid and could not be bent. It was used in the observation and research of skin and cervical and abdominal organs, and so on (Fig. 1.2). However, this type of confocal laser endomicroscope could not be used for the examination of the human gastrointestinal tract.[3]

At the beginning of this century, Optiscan Company and Pentax Company joined forces to develop CLE techniques. The use of ultraminiaturization technology made possible the development of a small-sized confocal laser scanner and optical image device (diameter 6 mm, length 70 mm) such that they could be integrated into the forefront of conventional endomicroscopy. A perfect combination of a confocal laser microscope with a conventional endomicroscope was completed and the flexible confocal laser endomicroscope was invented (Fig. 1.3).

Since 2003, this flexible confocal laser endomicroscope has been used in clinical trials, and has been shown to be effective in the examination of human colon diseases and upper gastrointestinal diseases

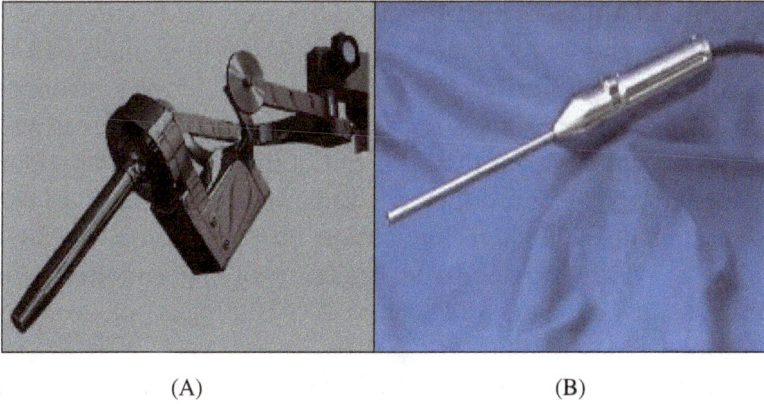

(A)   (B)

Fig. 1.2. Rigid confocal laser endomicroscopy. (A) The F900e rigid confocal laser endomicroscope invented in 1998. (B) The rigid confocal laser endomicroscope.

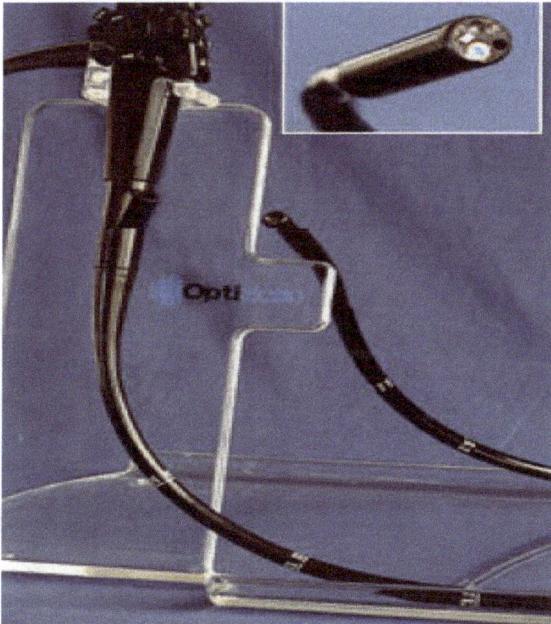

Fig. 1.3. Flexible confocal laser endomicroscopy.

in vivo in a number of clinical trials.[4] However, the front end of the confocal laser endomicroscope is about 70 mm long and cannot be bent, which impacts flexibility in the examination of the gastrointestinal tract. In recent years, the size of the confocal laser scanner as well as the optical image device at the front end of the confocal laser endomicroscope has been reduced further (diameter 5 mm, length 43 mm), thus making possible there integration into the Pentax EC3870K endoscope, which increased the flexibility of the endomicroscope (Fig. 1.4). The new endoscope, Pentax ISC-1000, was put into clinical application in March 2006.[5]

Recently, a kind of probe-based confocal laser endomicroscopy (pCLE) has been developed. Cellvizio® is a pCLE system that allows real-time microscopic imaging of the GI mucosa. The components of the system are the laser scanning unit, the processing station, and the Confocal Miniprobe,™ which is passed through the working channel of the endoscope. A range of miniprobes is available: GastroFlex™ and ColoFlex™ are designed for upper and lower luminal imaging through any gastroscope or colonoscope, and the ultrathin CholangioFlex™ miniprobe is dedicated to bile and pancreatic duct imaging through a cholangioscope or catheter (Figs. 1.5 and 1.6).[6,7]

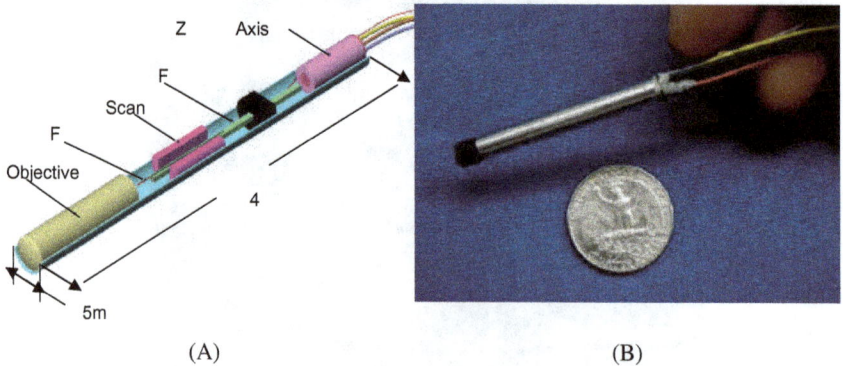

(A)   (B)

Fig. 1.4. The front-end of the Pentax ISC-1000 confocal laser endomicroscope. (A) The front end of the Pentax ISC-1000 confocal laser endomicroscope is further minimized to a diameter of 5 mm and a length of 43 mm. (B) Comparison of the size of a coin with the front end of the Pentax ISC-1000 confocal laser endomicroscope.

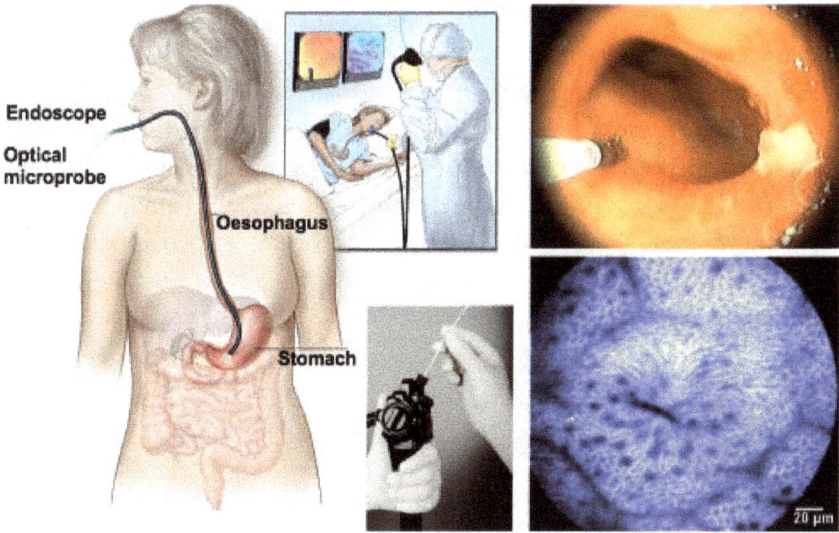

Fig. 1.5. The probe-based confocal laser endomicroscopy system.

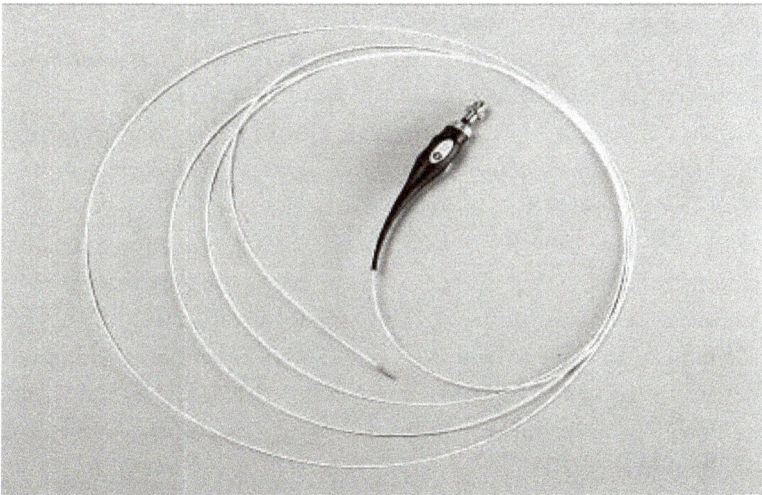

Fig. 1.6. Cellvizio® confocal laser endomicroscopy probe.

The Cellvizio® CLE probe can be put flexibly into the working channel of the ordinary endomicroscope, and can obtain microscopic imaging of the gastrointestinal mucosa in realtime.

CLE is a new tool that allows microscopic *in vivo* assessment of the GI mucosa. It is a revolutionary technology, providing endoscopists for the first time with information about living cells in human beings. We can carry out real-time "optical biopsy" in the process of gastrointestinal endoscopy through CLE. Despite the current limitations of CLE, such as scanning depth, scan area, and image quality, we believe that there will be further technical improvements and wider application of CLE in the near future.

References

1. Wright SJ, Wright DJ. (2002) Introduction to confocal microscopy. *Meth Cell Biol* **70**: 1–85.
2. Helmchen F. (2002) Miniaturization of fluorescence microscopes using fibre optics. *Exp Physiol* **87**(6): 737–745.
3. Polglase AL, McLaren WJ, Skinner SA, *et al.* (2005) A fluorescence confocal endomicroscope for *in vivo* microscopy of the upper- and the lower-GI tract. *Gastrointest Endosc* **62**(5): 686–695.
4. Kiesslich R, Goetz M, Vieth M, *et al.* (2005) Confocal laser endomicroscopy. *Gastrointest Endosc Clin N Am* **15**(4): 715–731.
5. Kiesslich R, Goetz M, Vieth M, *et al.* (2007) Technology insight: confocal laser endomicroscopy for *in vivo* diagnosis of colorectal cancer. *Nat Clin Pract Oncol* **4**(8): 480–490.
6. Wang TD, Friedland S, Sahbaie P, *et al.* (2007) Functional imaging of colonic mucosa with a fibered confocal microscope for realtime *in vivo* pathology. *Clin Gastroenterol Hepatol* **5**(1): 1300–1305.
7. Meining A, Saur D. Bajbouj M, *et al.* (2007) *In vivo* histopathology for detection of gastrointestinal neoplasia with a portable, confocal miniprobe: an examiner blinded analysis. *Clin Gastroenterol Hepatol* **5**(11): 1261–1267.

Part 2

INTRODUCTION

Chapter 2

The Technique of Confocal Laser Endomicroscopy

Confocal laser endomicroscopy (CLE) is the fusion of endoscopy and confocal microscopy. This technology, currently available, is either integrated into a flexible endoscope (CLE, such as Pentax EC-3870CILK/CIK) or a probe-based system that can be passed through the working channel of an endoscope (pCLE, such as Cellvizio). They have different depths of imaging, fields of view, and lateral resolutions (Table 2.1). We focus mainly on the confocal microscope integrated into the distal tip of a conventional upper endoscope, which enables simultaneous white-light endoscopy and confocal microscopy.

Table 2.1. Specifications of the Confocal Laser Endoscope

Type	EC-3870
Angle of view for endoscopic image (°)	140
Field of view for confocal image (μm)	475 × 475
Focus: Conventional endoscopic image (mm)	3–100
Confocal image (μm)	0–250
Deflection (°): Up/down	130/130
Right/left	120/120
Insertion tube (mm)	12.8
Instrument channel (mm)	2.8
Working length (mm)	1050/1300/1500/1700
Scanning rates (frames/sec): Faster	1.6 frames/sec (1024 × 512 pixels)
Slower	0.8 frames/sec (1024 × 1024 pixels)
Slice thickness (μm)	7
Lateral resolution (μm)	0.7

Components of the Confocal Laser Endomicroscope

Take the Pentax EC3870K, for example. In addition to the endomicroscope, the system encompasses a touchscreen monitor for the endomicrocopic image, a monitor for the endoscopic image, a video processor, a confocal optical unit, and a confocal control unit (Fig. 2.1).

The diameters of the distal tip and the insertion tube are 12.8 mm. Distal tip angulation is 130° for up/down movement and 120° for right/left movement. The distal tip of the confocal laser endomicroscope contains a confocal scanning microscope, an air and water jet

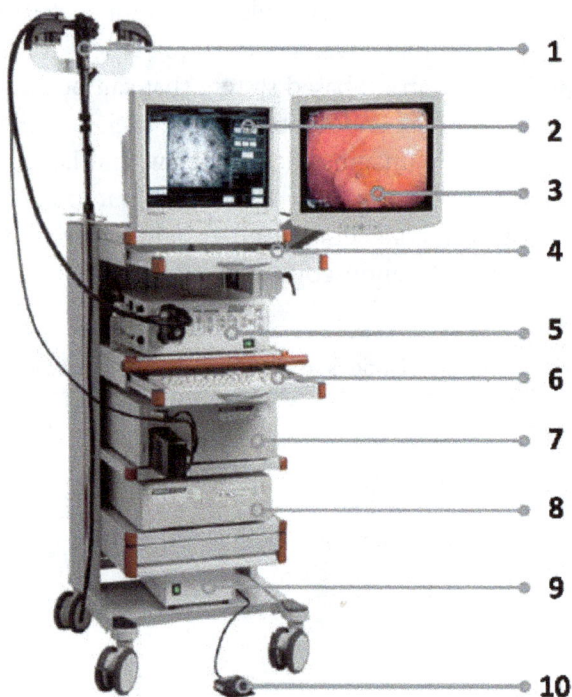

Fig. 2.1. The confocal laser endomicroscopy system. It comprises an endomicroscope (1), a touchscreen monitor for the endomicrocopic image (2), a monitor for the endoscopic image (3), a keyboard for the video processor (4), a video processor (5), a keyboard for the endomicroscopic system (6), a confocal optical unit (7), a confocal control unit (8), an isolation transformer (9), and a foot switch (10).

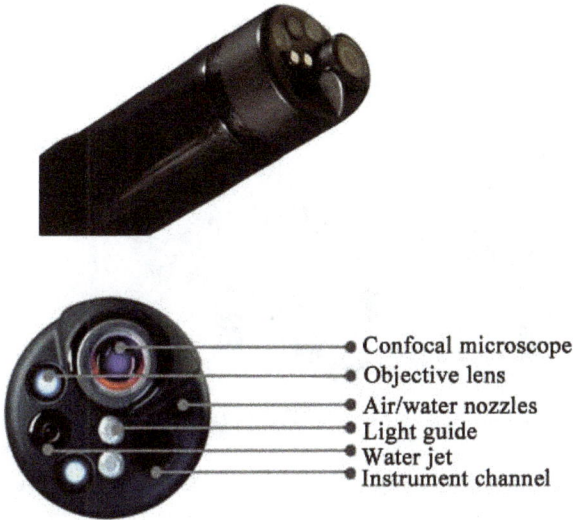

Fig. 2.2. The distal tip of the confocal laser endomicroscope. The confocal laser endoscope has a short protrusion at the distal tip, which contains the confocal microscope. Gentle contact with the mucosal surface is necessary in order to obtain microscopic images.

nozzle, two light guides, an auxiliary water jet channel (used for topical application of the contrast agent), and a 2.8 mm working channel (Fig. 2.2).[1] Actuation of the imaging plane depth is controlled by two additional handpiece buttons on the endoscope's control, the left button for resetting to the home position and the right button for control of the scanning depth (Fig. 2.3). Besides the control head, various scanning functions of the endomicroscope can be controlled using the touchscreen or keyboard mouse, such as the scanning rate, laser power, image brightness, and gamma settings (Fig. 2.4). The nonconfocal functionality of the endoscope tip of the confocal laser endomicroscope is comparable with that of a normal endoscope.

The confocal system has an additional optical unit and computer unit. During confocal laser endoscopy, a solid state ion laser delivers an excitation wavelength of 488 nm, and the maximum laser power output is <1 mw at the surface of the tissue. The optical slice thickness is 7 μm, with a lateral resolution of 0.7 μm (field of view 475 × 475 μm).

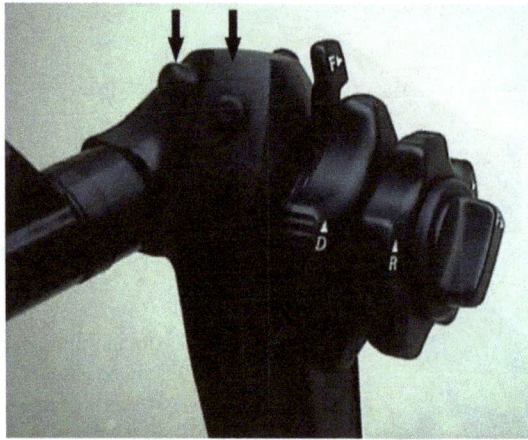

Fig. 2.3.   Control buttons of the confocal laser endomicroscope. The right button is used to reset to the home position and the left button is for control of scanning. One click of the left button causes the confocal imaging direction to return to the home position. The left button is used all the time during endomicroscopic imaging to move the scanning direction one plane up (two clicks) or down (one click).

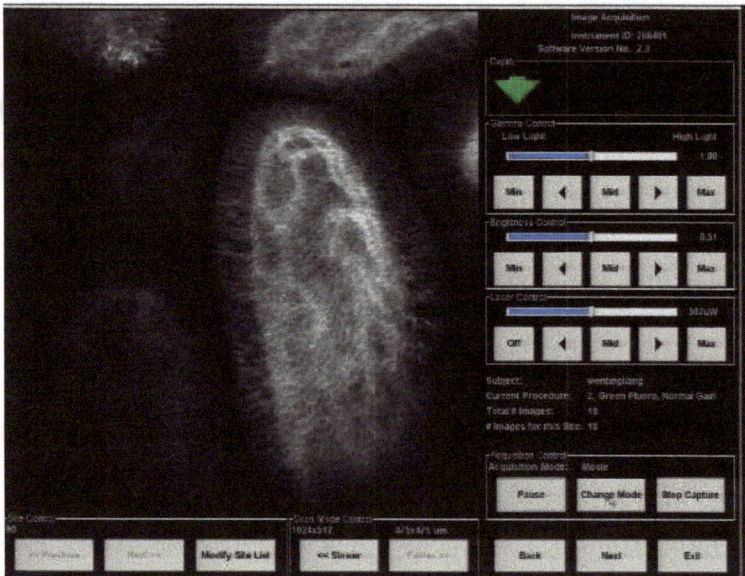

Fig. 2.4.   The control screen of confocal laser endomicroscopy. The default settings for the laser power, brightness, and gamma settings are all in the midposition.

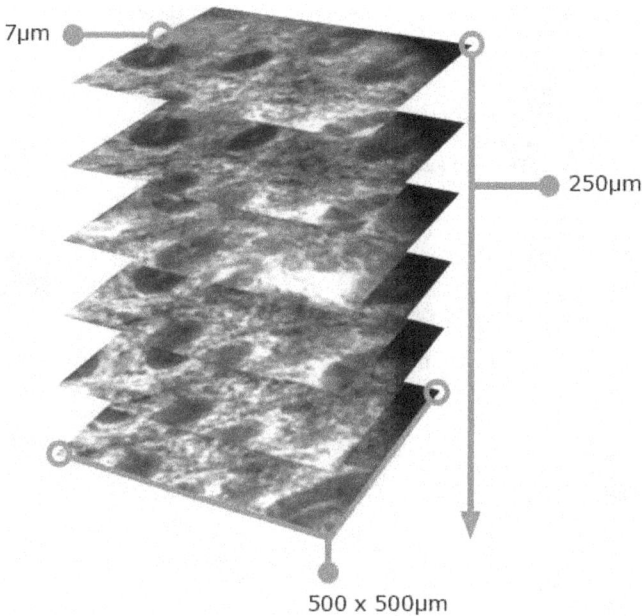

7μm

250μm

500 x 500μm

Fig. 2.5. Optical slices from the confocal laser endomicroscope.

The range of the z axis is 0–250 μm below the surface layer (Fig. 2.5). The confocal image data are collected at scanning rates of 1.6 frames/ sec (faster mode, 1024 × 512 pixels) or 0.8 frames/sec (slower mode, 1024 × 1024 pixels).

Basic Principle of Confocal Microscopy

Clinical endomicroscopy is an extension of conventional laboratory confocal microscopy. Confocal microscopy has become an essential tool for a wide range of investigations in the biological and medical sciences. It offers several advantages over conventional light microscopy, including the ability to control the depth of field, reduction in background information away from the focal plane, and the capability to obtain serial optical sections from specimens.[2,3]

The confocal principle of the laser scanning microscope is diagrammatically presented in Fig. 2.6. Coherent light emitted by the

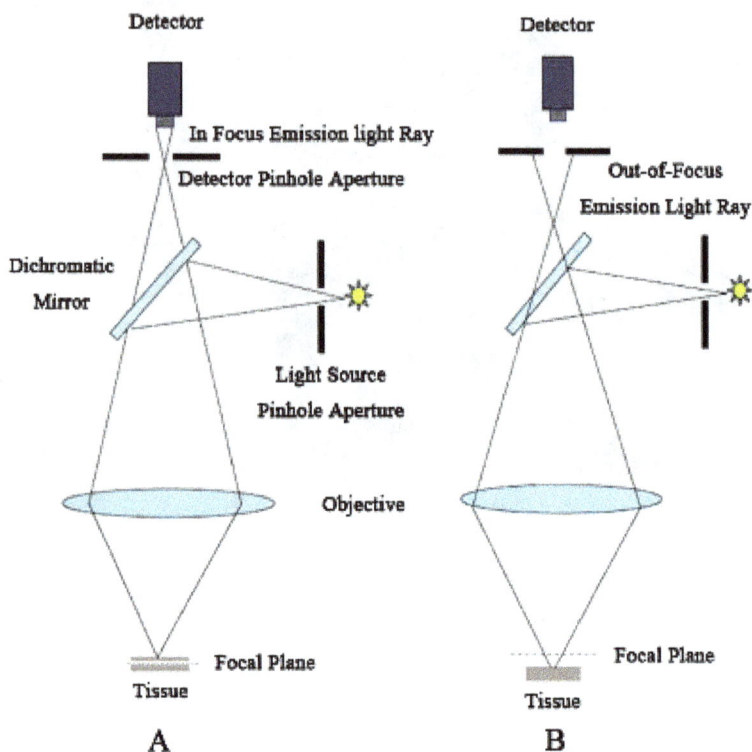

Fig. 2.6.   The principle of confocal microscopy.

laser excitation source passes through a pinhole that is situated in a conjugate plane with a scanning point on the specimen and a second pinhole positioned in front of the detector ("confocal" means that the light source pinhole, the scanning point of the specimen, and the detector pinhole are at the same focal plane). As the laser is reflected by a dichromatic mirror and scanned across the specimen in a defined focal plane, secondary fluorescence emitted from points on the specimen (in the same focal plane) pass back through the dichromatic mirror and are focused as a confocal point at the detector pinhole (Fig. 2.6A).

But the fluorescence emission that occurs at points above and below the objective focal plane is not confocal with the pinhole and only forms extended Airy disks in the detector pinhole plane. Therefore, most of this extraneous light can not be detected and does not contribute to the resulting image (Fig. 2.6B).

Endomicroscopy and confocal microscopy share the same principle. The development of technology makes it possible to use an optical fiber to transmit the laser from its source to illuminate a specimen, and the same optical fiber can then be used to carry the return light back to an image acquisition system. Meanwhile, the use of flexible optical fiber allows endomicroscopy to separate the large laser and control systems from the microscope's scanning head (Fig. 2.7).[4] Blue laser light is focused on the desired tissue via the distal tip, applied fluorescent contrast agents are excited by the laser lights, and the special confocal optical unit exclusively detects the fluorescing light at a defined horizontal level (Fig. 2.8).[5]

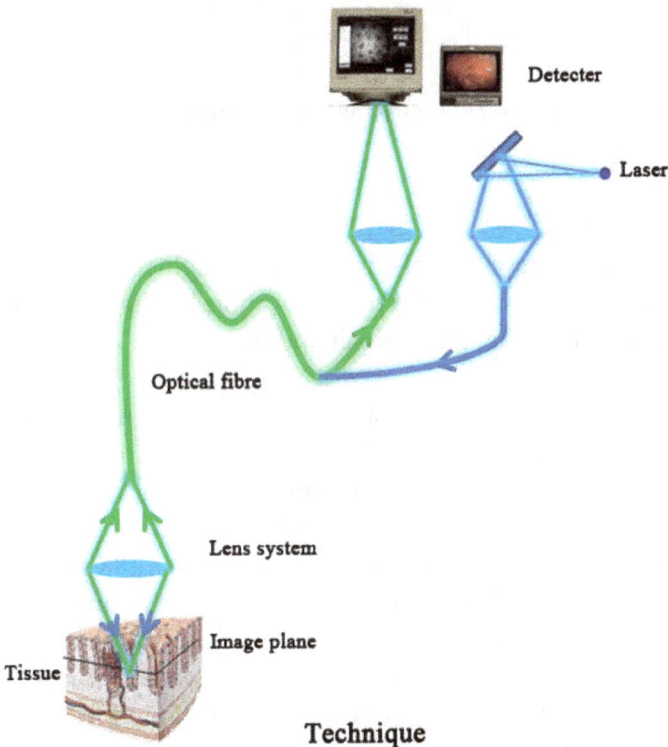

Fig. 2.7. Optical scheme of endomicroscopy.

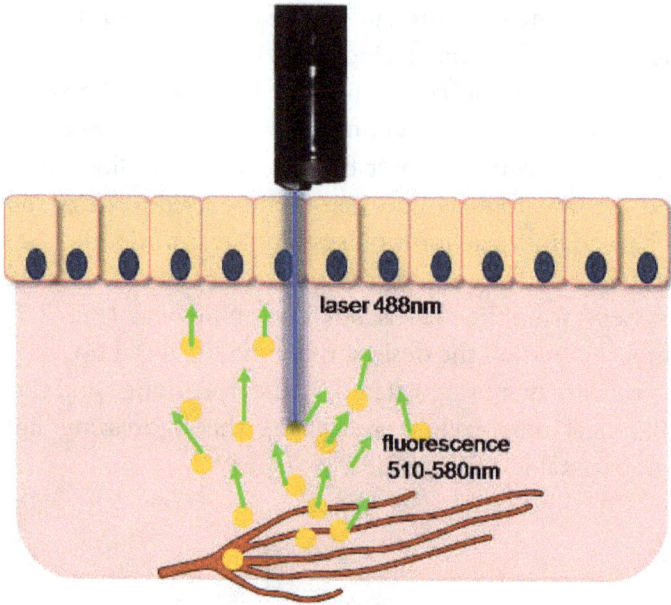

Fig. 2.8. Fluorescent contrast agents are excited by the laser light.

Contrast Agents

Contrast agents are essential for achieving high resolution confocal images. They can be administered intravenously (fluorescein sodium) or topically (acriflavine, cresyl violet and tetracycline) through a spraying catheter.

The most common contrast agent used so far is fluorescein sodium (10% solution, 5–10 ml). Fluorescein sodium is inexpensive and nonmutagenic, and has been safely used for decades in ophthalmology in human beings. Fluorescein absorbs light in the blue range of the visible spectrum, with absorption peaking at 488 nm (blue) and emission peaking at 530 nm (yellow).[6,7] Because the current CLE system uses a single detector, the CLE image is in black and white, and the fluorescein signal shows white in the confocal image. Approximately 70%–80% of fluorescein will be bound to plasma albumin after injection; then it is transmitted through the circulatory system to mucosal capillaries, and unbound fluorescein (20%–30%)

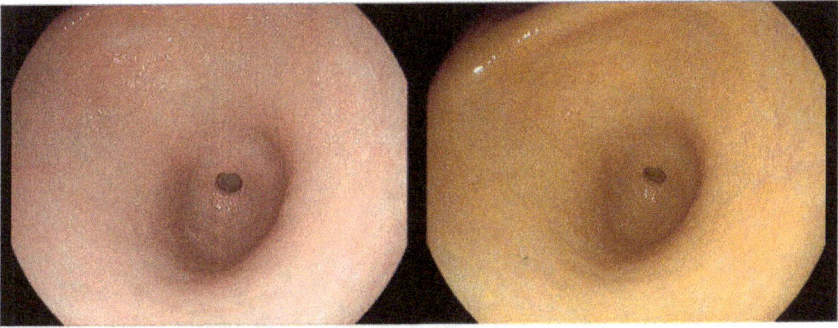

Fig. 2.9. Yellow discoloration of the mucosa after administration of fluorescein.

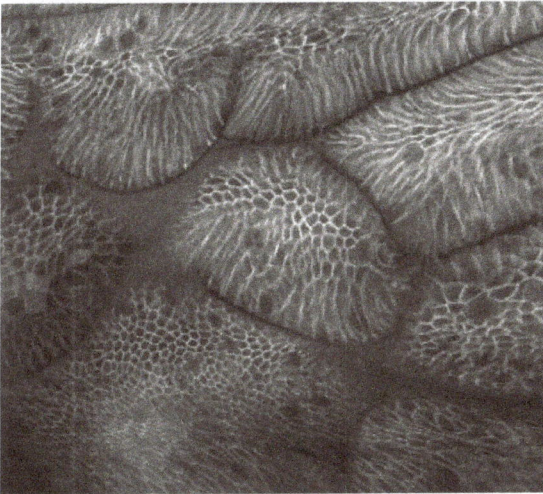

Fig. 2.10. CLE images after administration of fluorescein. Goblet cells appear dark within the columnar epithelium because mucin is not stained by fluorescein.

can leak from the capillaries and is distributed throughout the entire mucosa with a strong contrast within the connective tissue and the capillary network (Figs. 2.9–2.11).[8] However, cell nuclei and mucin are not stained by fluorescein and therefore appear dark (Fig. 2.12).

CLE images can be obtained from about 15 s after intravenous injection for up to 30 min. Elimination is predominantly renal but

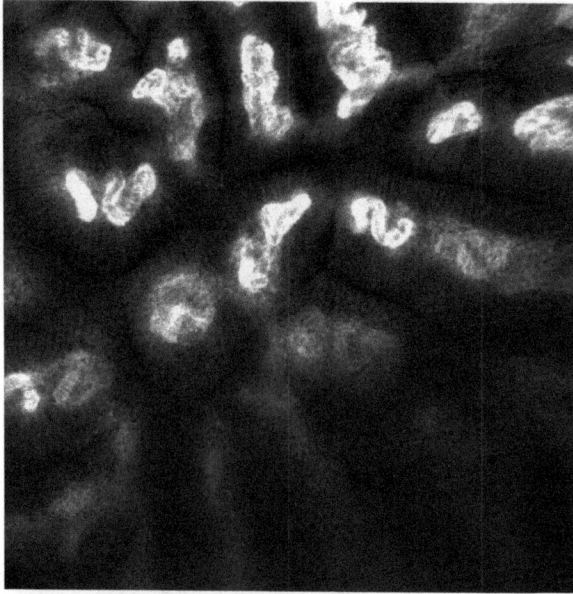

Fig. 2.11. CLE images after administration of fluorescein. Fluorescein can leak from the capillaries with a strong contrast within the connective tissue and the capillary network.

also via the liver and in the feces. One-time dosage of fluorescein is excreted almost completely within 48 h after administration. The safety of intravenous fluorescein is well established for its use in ophthalmological angiography. Transient yellow discoloration of the skin and urine is common with the use of fluorescein. Severe adverse reactions such as shock, thrombophlebitis, and anaphylaxis are rare.[9] Mild adverse events include nausea, vomiting, transient hypotension, diffuse rash, and mild epigastric pain.[10]

Topically administered contrast agents are applied on the surface of the mucosa by using a spraying catheter after mucolysis. Acriflavine hydrochloride (0.05% solution) can be highly specific for labeling acidic constituents and stains the nuclei.[4] Therefore, acriflavine is very useful for identifying intraepithelial neoplasia and cancer of the GI tract. But the imaging depth is limited to the surface layers of the mucosa (down to a depth of 100 µm) (Figs. 2.13 and 2.14).

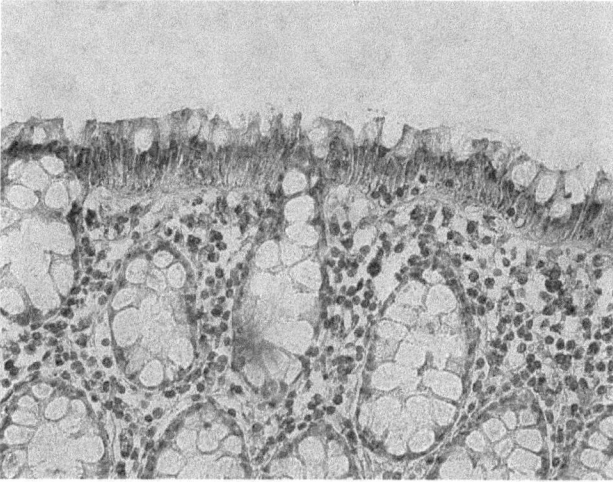

Fig. 2.12. Antifluorescein antibody staining by immunohistochemistry. The immunohistochemical localization of fluorescein was consistent with the CLE images. No staining was observed in the nucleus and mucin of goblet cells.

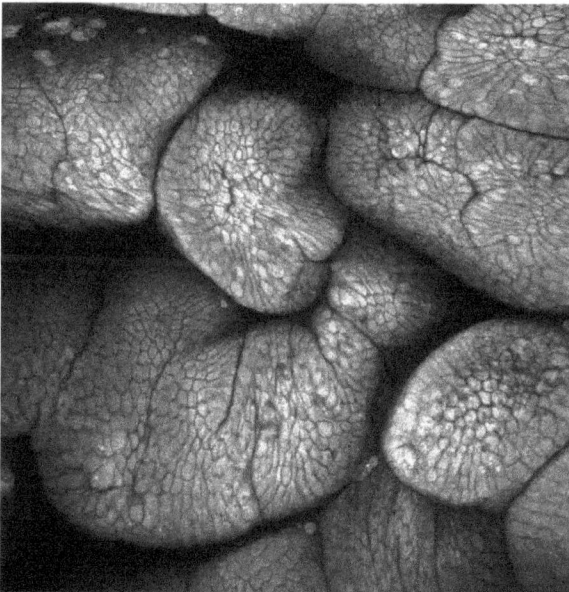

Fig. 2.13. CLE images after administration of acriflavine. The imaging depth is limited to the surface layers of the mucosa.

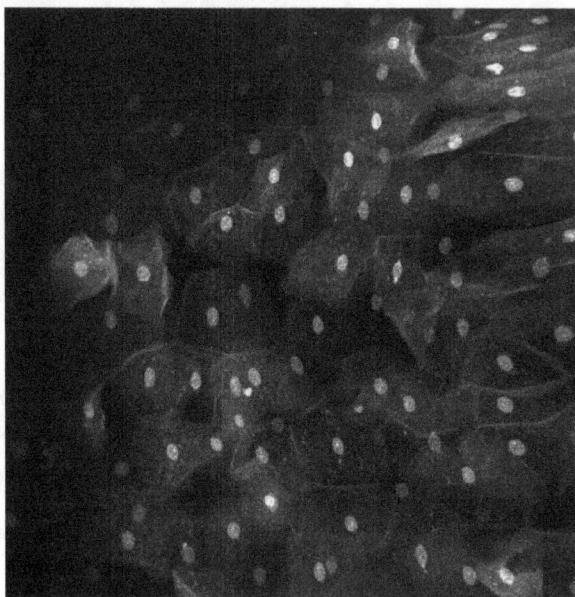

Fig. 2.14.   CLE images after administration of acriflavine. The staining provides clear visualization of cell nuclei in the surface mucosa.

Up to now no severe adverse reactions have been reported after the topical use of acriflavine.[11]

Crystal violet is an absorptive coloring agent and has been applied in chromoendoscopy for enhancing visualization of the pit patterns. 0.05%–0.2% crystal violet solution was previously used and Goetz *et al.* suggested that a concentration as low as 0.13% was adequate for endomicroscopy.[12,13] The staining technique is similar to that for acriflavine. However, by cytoplasmic enrichment of crystal violet, the nuclear morphology was negatively visualized as dark areas on the basal side of the epithelial cells.

Clinical Procedures

The preparations for CLE observation are similar to those for conventional endoscopy. It is contraindicated in people with asthma or a known allergy to fluorescein, impaired renal function, pregnancy, and breastfeeding. Patients need to be given intravenous injections of 1 ml of 2% fluorescein sodium for an allergy test before the procedures. If necessary, the mucosal surface can be treated with a mucolytic agent, such as chymotrypsin or N-acetylcysteine. When we turn on the endomicroscopy software, the program is first self-explanatory, case information will be entered, and specific sites may be chosen and moved to the "selected sites" list on the left of the screen.

The confocal endoscope can be handled in a similar way to a standard endoscope. After the standard endoscopy procedure, contrast agents are applied intravenously or topically. Then you should shift your focus from the endoscopic image to the endomicroscopic image displayed on the other monitor. Make sure that the laser is turned on by choosing the default midposition. The endomicroscopic image is acquired by placing the tip of the colonoscope in gentle contact with the target tissue site. The direct scanning plane is evident by the laser raster, which is visible on the target mucosal site as a blue scanning beam at the lower-left corner (Fig. 2.15). If

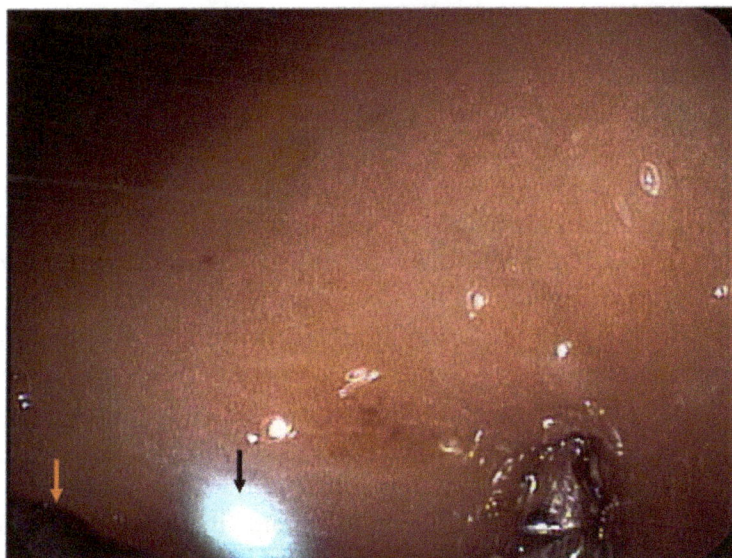

Fig. 2.15. The distal tip of the endoscope (*orange arrow*) and the laser raster (*black arrow*) are visible at the lower-left corner.

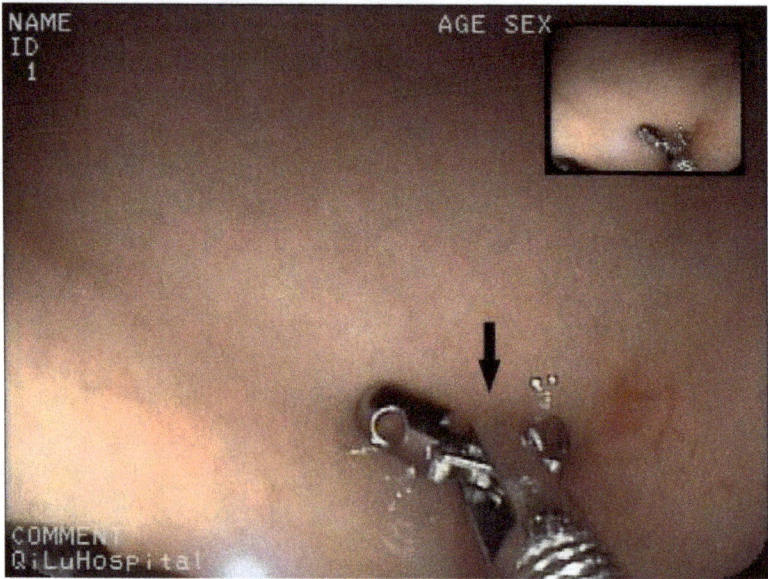

Fig. 2.16.   The "optical biopsy" site.

gentle pressure does not result in an adequate stable image, we can apply suction to maintain a stable position. However, observation sites of the fundus and cardia are difficult to investigate, due to the limitation of angulation.

The "optical biopsy" site was located 5 mm immediately to the left of the erythema created by suction using conventional white light imaging (Fig. 2.16). The site of interest in the mucosal layer could be scanned from the surface to the deeper areas. Each click resulted in a 10–15 μm change of the scanning depth, and images could be captured by operating a foot pedal. If the image appears too bright or too dark, make adjustments of the laser power button to optimize the images.

Motion artefact and contamination are the main artefact during imaging. Sometimes it is difficult to obtain fine images because of mucosal movement caused by the heartbeat, respiration, and peristalsis. Endoscope movement and tip movement can also cause motion

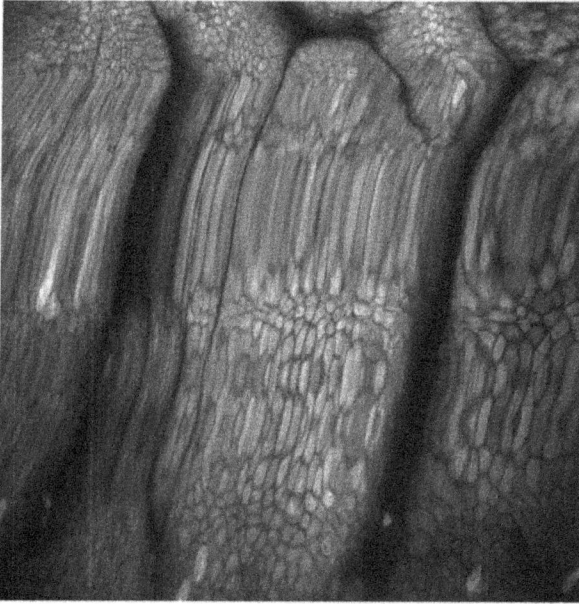

Fig. 2.17.   Motion artefact. It appears as blurring and ghosting of images.

artefact (Fig. 2.17). It is more commonly seen in the upper gastrointestinal tract, especially in the esophagus and cardia. It is reduced in anesthetized patients during endoscopy, and we can capture confocal images using the faster rate (1.6 frames/sec) to diminish this influence.

A contamination image can be caused by mucus, blood, extravasated fluorescein, food, or stool on the confocal lens. It has various kinds of manifestation, such as bright or dark splotches. However, when we capture confocal images dynamically, the contamination splotches will usually not change their location on the monitor. This feature can distinguish contamination from goblet cells, gaps, or other mucosal architectures (Fig. 2.18). It is necessary to avoid bleeding from the lesions (tumor, ulcer, or IBD) due to abrasion by the tip of the endoscope. Areas can be washed with water if details are obscured by mucus.

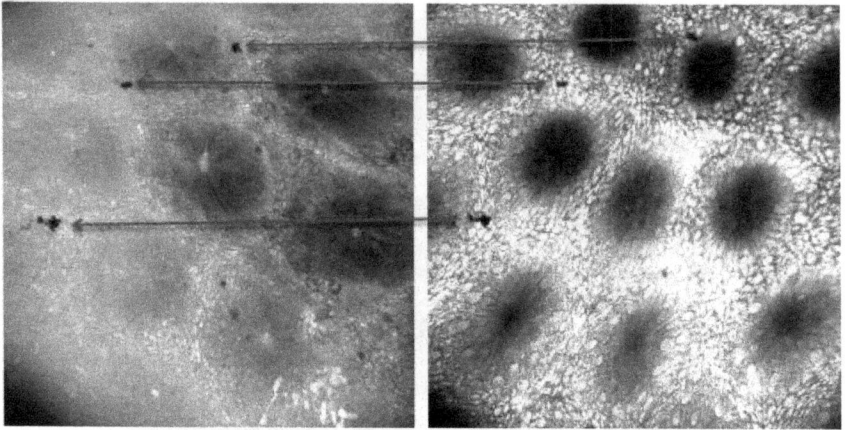

Fig. 2.18.   Contamination image. The contamination splotches will not change when we capture the confocal images dynamically.

References

1. Hoffman A, Goetz M, Vieth M, *et al.* (2006) Confocal laser endomicroscopy: technical status and current indications. *Endoscopy* **38**: 1275–1283.
2. Müller M. (2002) *Introduction to Confocal Fluorescence Microscopy*. Shaker, Maastricht.
3. Hibbs AR. (2004) *Confocal Microscopy for Biologists*. Kluwer Academic, New York.
4. Polglase AL, McLaren WJ, Skinner SA, *et al.* (2005) A fluorescence confocal endomicroscope for *in vivo* microscopy of the upper- and the lower-GI tract. *Gastrointest Endosc* **62**: 686–695.
5. Yoshida S, Tanaka S, Hirata M, *et al.* (2007) Optical biopsy of GI lesions by reflectance-type laser-scanning confocal microscopy. *Gastrointest Endosc* **66**: 144–149.
6. Selkin B, Rajadhyaksha M, Gonzalez S, *et al.* (2001) *In vivo* confocal microscopy in dermatology. *Dermatol Clin* **19**: 369–377.
7. Kim J. (2007) The use of vital dyes in corneal disease. *Curr Opin Ophthalmol* **11**: 241–247.
8. Pawley JB. (2002) Limitations on optical sectioning in live-cell confocal microscopy. *Scanning* **24**: 241–246.

9. Jennings BJ, Matthews DE. (1994) Adverse reactions during retinal fluorescein angiography. *J Am Optom Assoc* **65**: 465–471.

10. Moosbrugger KA, Sheidow TG. (2008) Evaluation of the side effects and image quality during fluorescein angiography comparing 2 mL and 5 mL sodium fluorescein. *Can J Ophthalmol* **43**: 571–575.

11. Hurlstone DP, Brown S. (2007) Techniques for targeting screening in ulcerative colitis. *Postgrad Med J* **83**: 451–460.

12. Kudo S, Rubio CA, Teixeira CR, *et al.* (2001) Pit pattern in colorectal neoplasia: endoscopic magnifying view. *Endoscopy* **33**: 367–373.

13. Goetz M, Toermer T, Vieth M, *et al.* (2009) Simultaneous confocal laser endomicroscopy and chromoendoscopy with topical cresyl violet. *Gastrointest Endosc* **70**: 959–968.

Part 3

ESOPHAGUS

Chapter 3

Normal Esophagus and Endomicroscopic Imaging

Normal Esophageal Mucosa

The adult esophagus is a muscular tube some 25 cm long, extending from the pharynx to the cardia. The wall of the esophagus contains four layers, from inner to outer: mucosa, submucosa, tunica muscularis, and tunica adventitia.

The mucosa is some 500–800 μm thick and is composed of epithelium with subjacent lamina propria and the underlying muscularis mucosae. Of these, the epithelial thickness is about 260–440 μm.[1]

The esophageal epithelium is not completely keratinized stratified squamous epithelium, but consists of a variable number of cell layers transiting from the cuboidal basal layer to the more flattened surface layer. In the transitional process, specific cell layers have formed: basal layer, spinosum layer, granular layer, and nonkeratinized superficial layer. The proliferation and regeneration of the esophageal epithelium are due to mitosis of the basal cells. As the cells migrate toward the lumen, they become gradually polygonal and more flattened, and are eventually desquamated at the epithelial surface.

Usually, the basal layer is the deepest cell layer of the epithelium. The basal cells are cuboidal or oblong and relatively small, with larger global nuclei lying on the basement and hyperbasophilic plasma. The cells overlying the basal cells, the stratum spinosum, are polygonal and contain some 3–8 layers of cells, with larger nuclei and less hyperchromatic plasma compared to the basal cells.

31

As cells approach the apical layer of the squamous epithelium, they become bigger and flattened, with increasingly elliptical nuclei transiting toward the cell surface, and less hyperchromatic plasma; this layer is called the granular layer. In the most superficial layer of the esophageal epithelium, the cells are flattened but retain their nuclei, which indicates that the squamous epithelium is not completely keratinized (Figs. 3.1–3.8).

The esophageal lamina propria is loose connective tissue, containing capillaries, lymphatic channels, elastic fibers and in some instances, inflammatory cells. The short indentations of soft tissue in the squamous epithelium are called epithelial papillae, which enlarge the contact area between the epithelium and the lamina propria.

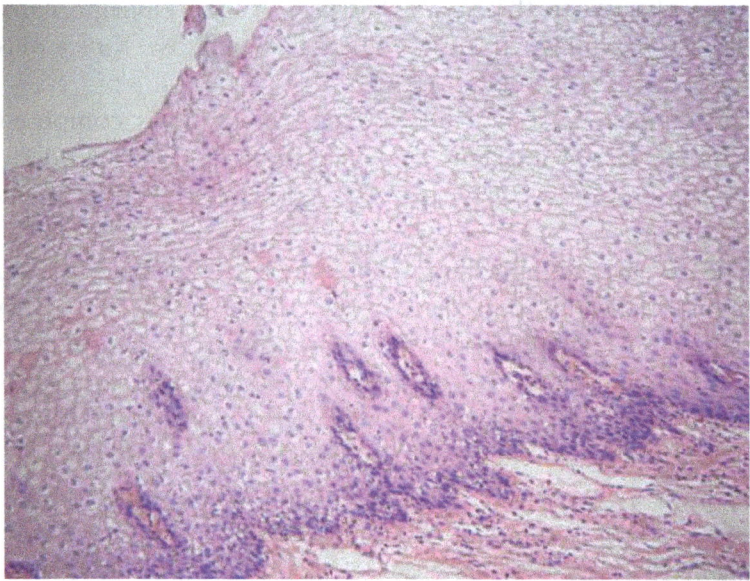

Fig. 3.1.   Esophageal epithelium (vertical section) HE × 100. Change in the shapes of esophageal squamous epithelial layers. The basal cells are relatively small, with larger global nuclei lying on the basement and hyperbasophilic plasma. As the cells migrate toward the lumen, they become bigger and flattened, with increased elliptical nuclei transiting toward the cell surface, and lessened chromatic plasma. Even in the most superficial layer of the esophageal epithelium, the cells still retain their nuclei.

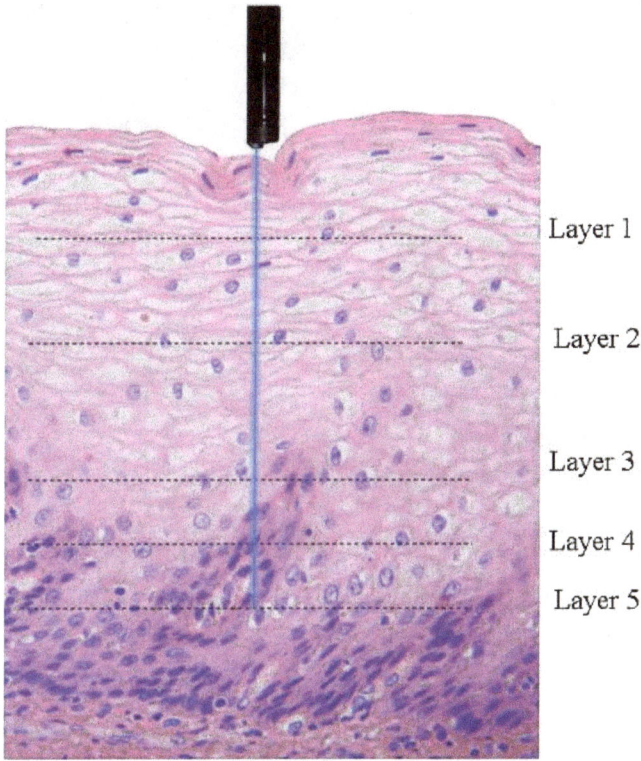

Layer 1

Layer 2

Layer 3

Layer 4

Layer 5

Fig. 3.2. Image showing the layers, respectively.

In normal conditions, these papillae are not elongated by more than 10%–20% of the total epithelial thickness.

Muscularis mucosa, which underlies the lamina propria, is the deepest portion of the esophageal mucosa, consisting of longitudinal smooth muscle bundles.

Endomicroscopic Imaging of Normal Esophageal Mucosa

With the assistance of suitable contrast agents, the cells and subcellular structures of the esophagus can be observed clearly by using CLE. Through the intravenous administration of 10% fluorescein sodium, it is possible to visualize whole depths of the esophageal epithelium,

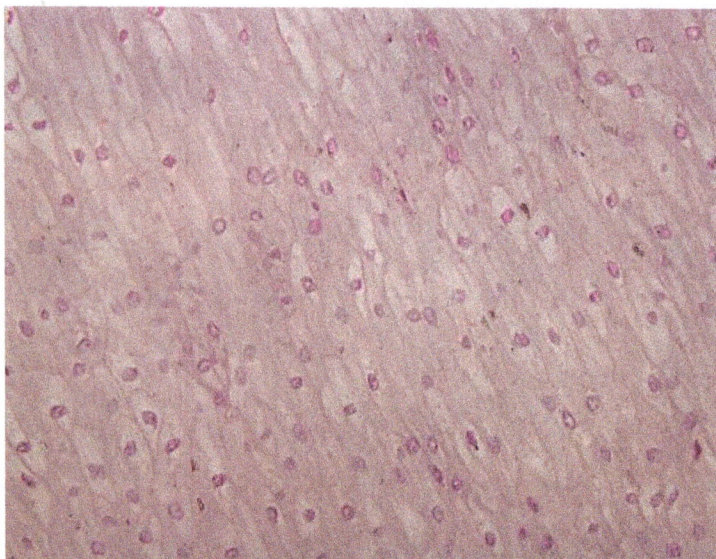

Fig. 3.3. The most superficial cross-section of squamous epithelium. The cells are bigger and more flattened, with concentrated nuclei (layer 1).

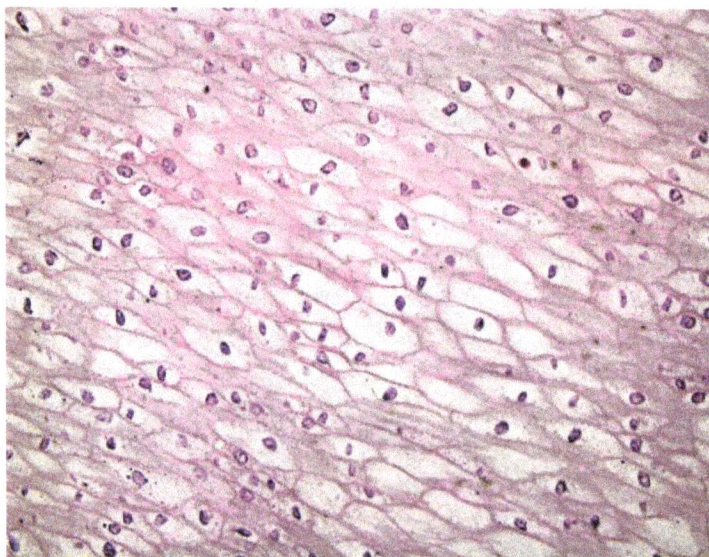

Fig. 3.4. The squamous epithelium of the esophagus. The papillae have not appeared yet, and the cells are flattened or fusiform (layer 2).

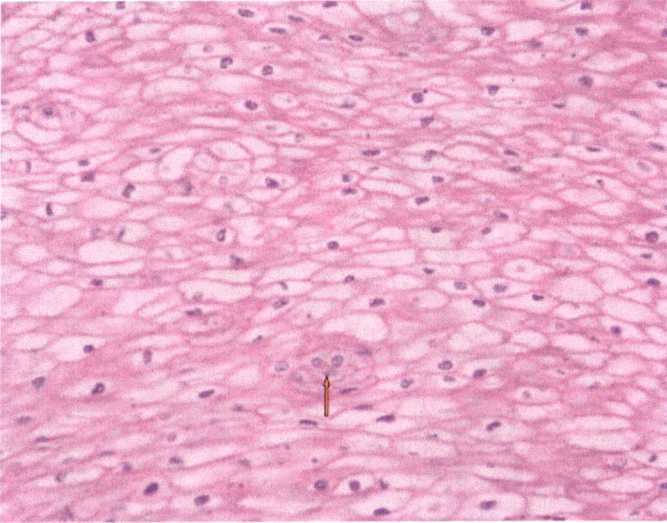

Fig. 3.5. Esophageal squamous epithelium. Polygonal cells (*arrow*) are visible which belong to the stratum spinosum and indicate the immediate appearance of papillae (layer 3).

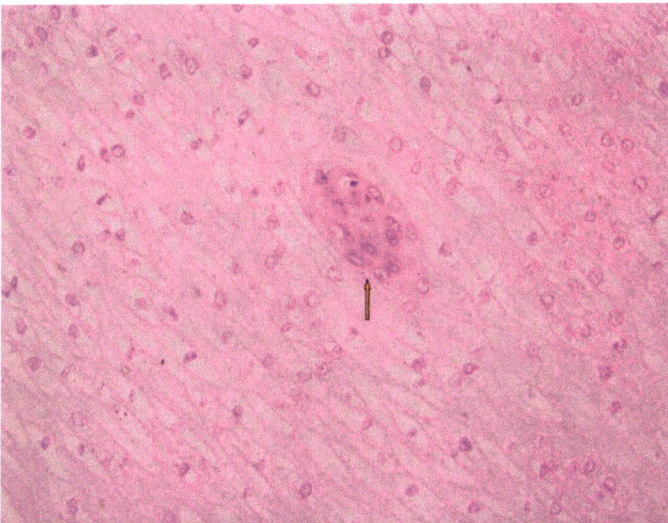

Fig. 3.6. Esophageal squamous epithelium and the papillae protruding from the lamina propria (*arrow*). The papillae have just appeared; their surroundings are basal cells and the outer ones are spinosum cells (layer 4).

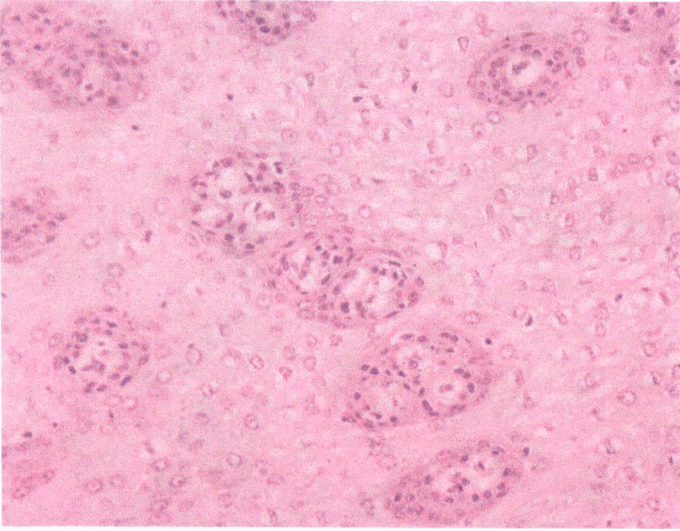

Fig. 3.7.   Esophageal squamous epithelium and papillae. The papillae have appeared and been in deeper gradation; their surroundings are basal cells. They have smaller bodies but bigger nuclei compared with the more superficial layer, and the plasma is basophilic (layer 5).

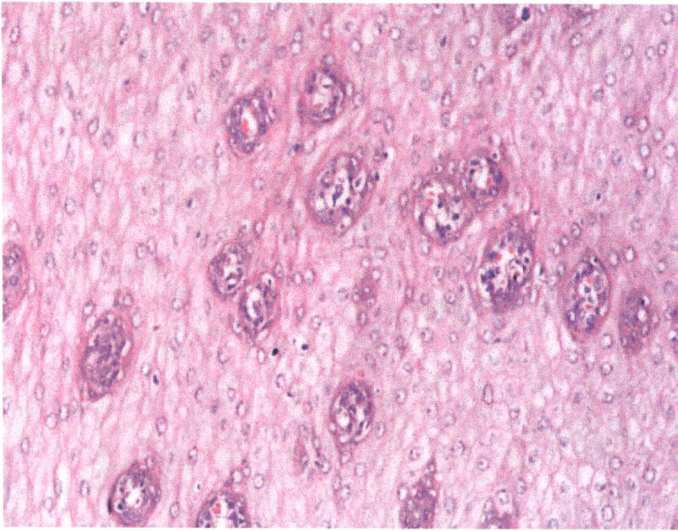

Fig. 3.8.   Esophageal squamous epithelium and papillae. The blood vessels in the lamina propria can be observed (layer 5).

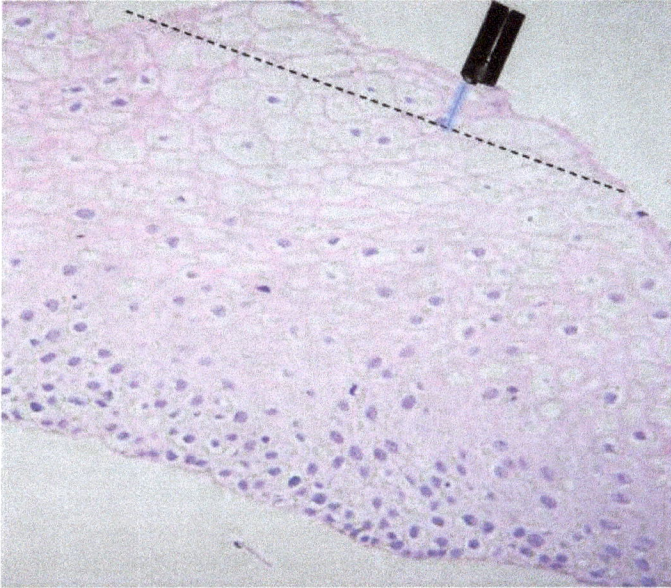

Fig. 3.9. Normal esophageal vertical-section image (HE × 200).

partial structures of the lamina propria, and the changes of intrapapillary capillary loops (IPCLs). Spraying 0.02% acriflavine on the luminal surface can highlight single squamous epithelial cells, especially nuclei, and the changes of cellular interspaces.

In endomicroscopic imaging of normal esophageal mucosa, the superficial planes are regularly arranged identical squamous epithelial cells, which have clear borders and a flattened nucleus. The cells surrounding the IPCLs are dense. The shapes of IPCLs change with the scanning depth, and the superficial squamous epithelium can be observed more clearly.

The cells of the nonkeratinized superficial layer, which lies on the surface of the epithelium, are derived from basal cells and contain no organellae. The concentrated nucleus contains many keratofilaments. The cellular junctions are rarely visualized (Figs. 3.9–3.11).

The cells of the stratum spinosum, which overlies the basal layer, are polygonal. The cells of the more superficial layer are increasingly

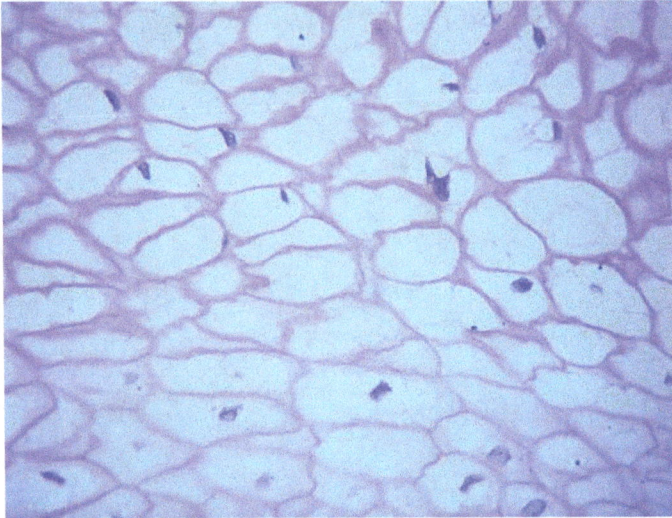

Fig. 3.10. Cross-section of the most superficial layer of the esophageal epithelium (HE × 400). The cells are flattened and the concentrated nuclei can be seen in partial cells.

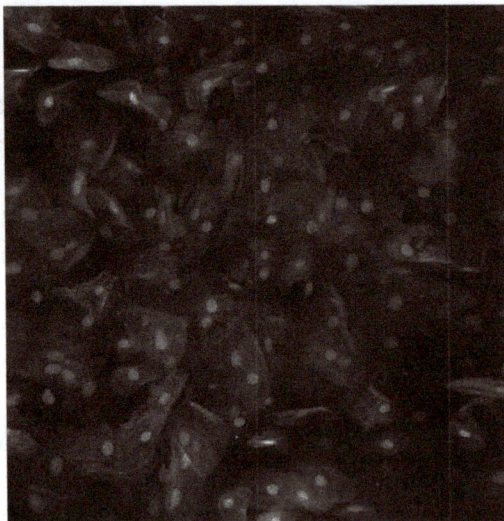

Fig. 3.11. After spraying 0.02% acriflavine on the luminal surface, it is possible to observe flattened squamous cells with distinct nuclei. The epithelial cells and their nuclei are uniform in shape.

flattened and less chromatic, whereas the cells of the deeper layer are intensely basophilic, the surroundings of which are the IPCLs projecting upward from the lamina propria (Figs. 3.12–3.15).

The basal layer is the deepest layer of the esophageal epithelium. CLE cannot scan the cells of the basal layer because of the thickness of the epithelium, but it is possible to observe the circle-like or short rod-like IPCLs with or without dilatation and squamous cells surrounding the IPCLs arranged in a concentric circle pattern (Figs. 3.16–3.19).

At the Z-line position, CLE can clearly distinguish the junction of esophageal squamous epithelium and cardiac columnar epithelium: the junctional line is distinct, and the columnar epithelial cells are uniform and regularly arranged, on whose side the gastric pits are mostly round or slightly irregular, but sparser and bigger than those in the gastric fundus and gastric body (Figs. 3.20–3.24).

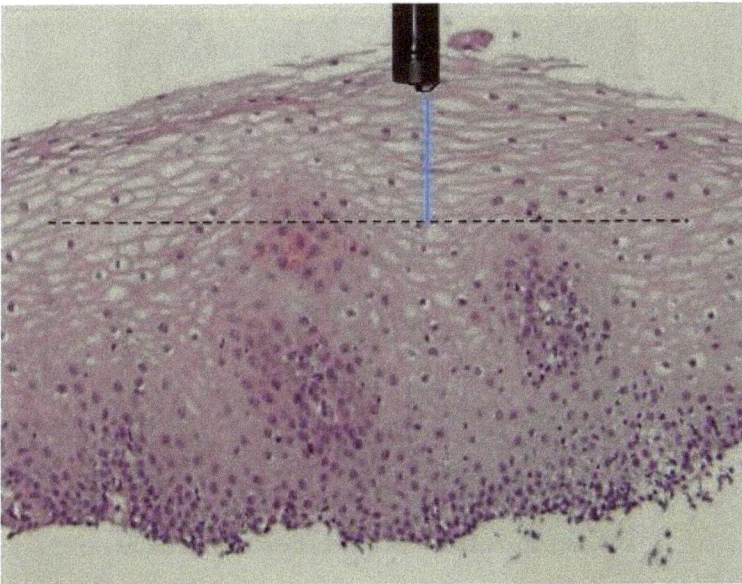

Fig. 3.12. Normal esophageal vertical-section image. The depth of this cross-section image is stratum spinosum.

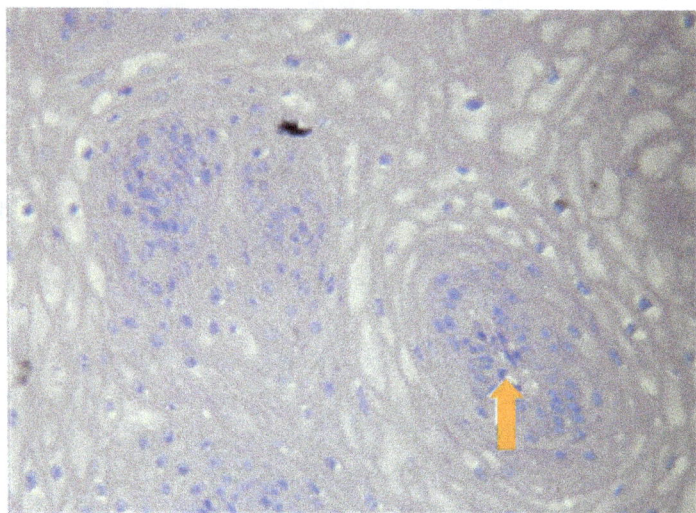

Fig. 3.13.   Cross-section of the esophageal epithelial spinosum layer (HE × 400). The cells are polygonal. The nuclei are bigger and less chromatic compared with the basal cells. The intrapapillary capillary loops (IPCLs) can be identified (arrow).

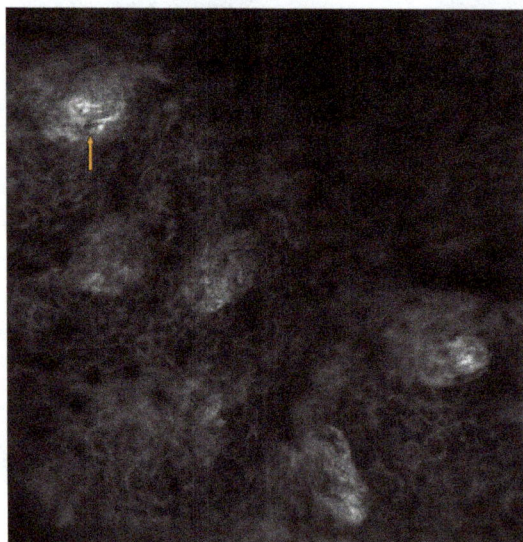

Fig. 3.14.   With the application of 10% fluorescein sodium, it is possible to observe the nuclei presenting black spots and distinct cellular interspaces. The apex of the IPCL can be seen (*arrow*).

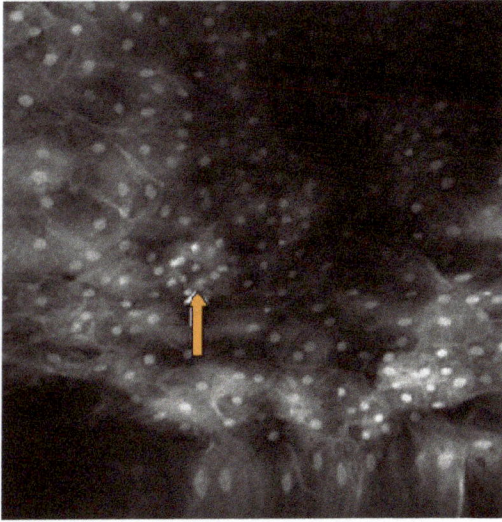

Fig. 3.15. After spraying 0.02% acriflavine on the luminal surface, the squamous cells become polygonal or fusiform, the cellular interspaces assume a distinct white line, and the nuclei are more concentrated than the keratinized layer. The dense light stack is the apex of the IPCL (*arrow*).

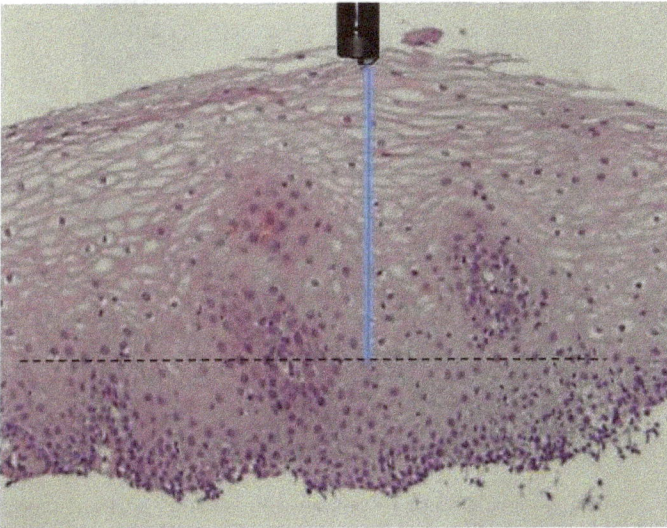

Fig. 3.16. Normal esophageal vertical-section image. The CLE scanning depth is the junction between the spinosum layer and the basal layer.

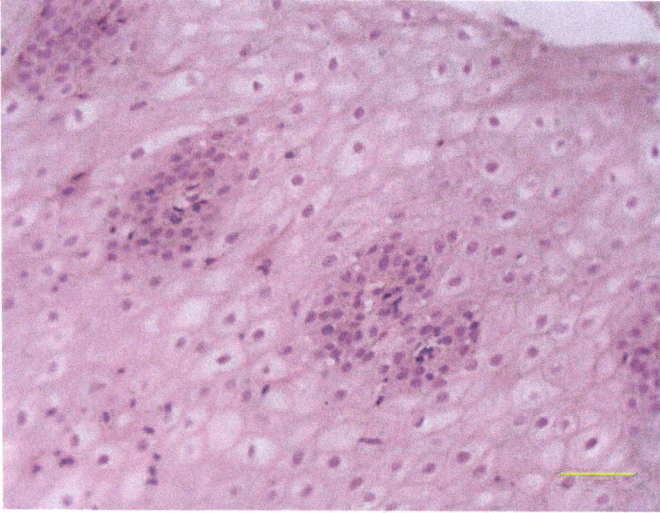

Fig. 3.17. The deeper part of the esophageal epithelial spinosum layer (HE × 400). The cells are polygonal. There are many IPCLs whose surroundings are basal squamous epithelial cells.

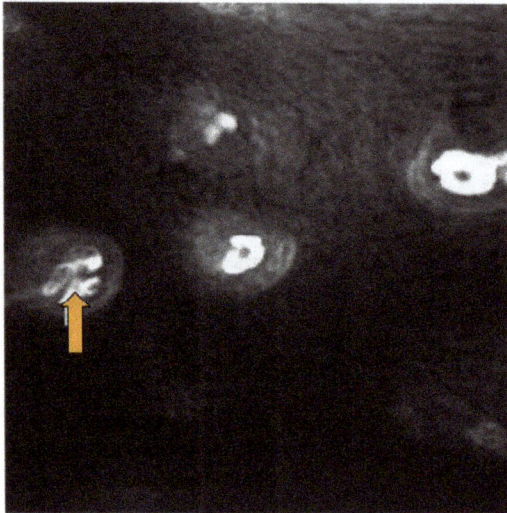

Fig. 3.18. With the application of 10% fluorescein sodium, IPCLs assume a circular or short rod-like appearance, with homogeneous calibers and no obvious dilatation. The surrounding squamous cells are arranged in a concentric circle pattern. Amidst the IPCLs are erythrocytes which look like black dots (*arrow*).

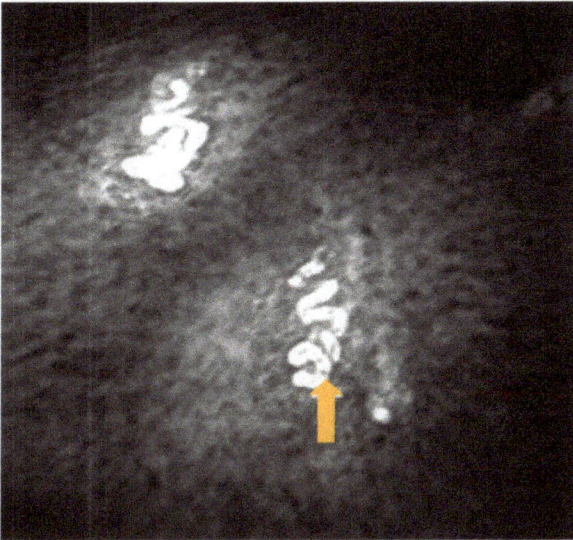

Fig. 3.19. With the application of 10% fluorescein sodium, IPCLs assume a circular appearance with equal calibers and no dilatation. Amidst the IPCLs are erythrocytes which look like black dots (*arrow*).

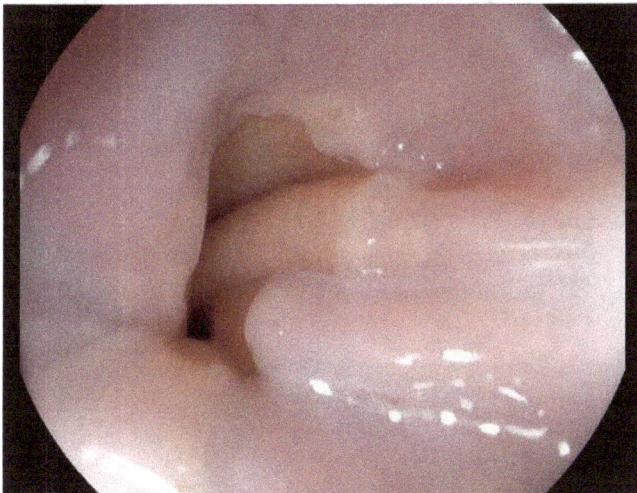

Fig. 3.20. Endoscopic imaging of the serrated line demarcated by esophageal mucosa and gastric mucosa. The superjacent is the pink esophageal mucosa, and the subjacent is the orange gastric mucosa.

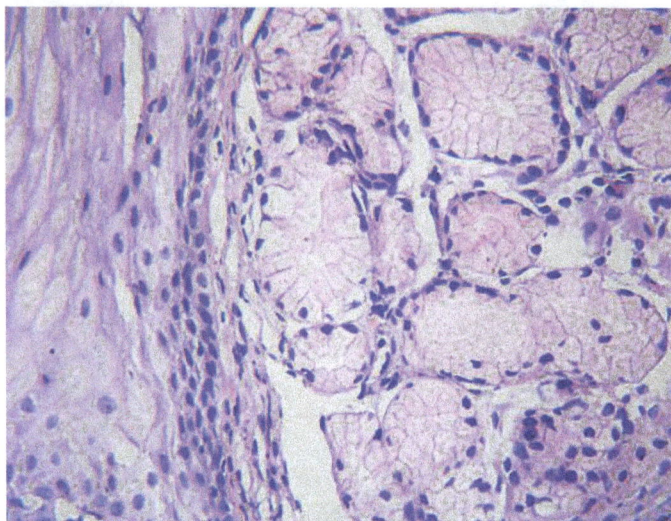

Fig. 3.21. The squamocolumnar junction in the distal esophagus (HE × 400). Cardiac glands have a larger glandular cavity; most are mucous glands, and do not contain chief cells and parietal cells.

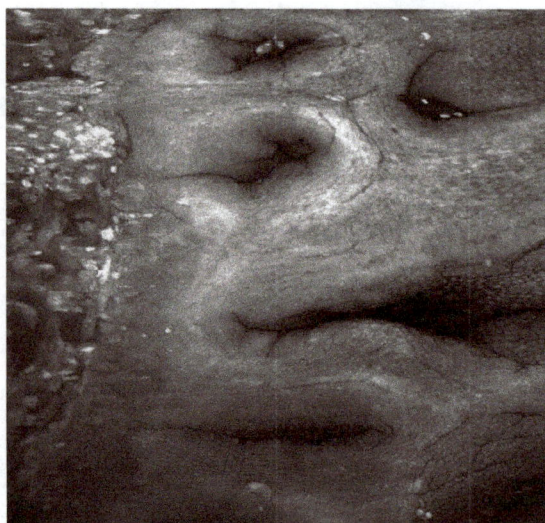

Fig. 3.22. The squamocolumnar junction after spraying 0.02% acriflavine. The junction of squamous epithelium and columnar epithelium is distinct, and the gastric pits are ovoid or irregular in shape.

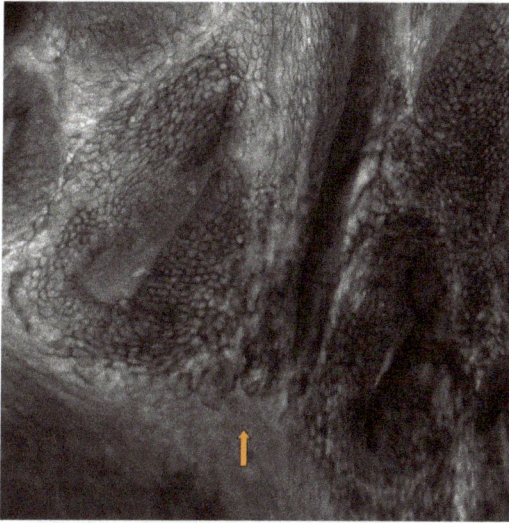

Fig. 3.23. With the administration of 10% fluorescein sodium. The arrow indicates the junction of squamous epithelium and columnar epithelium. On the columnar epithelial side, the glandular openings are ovoid (superficial layer).

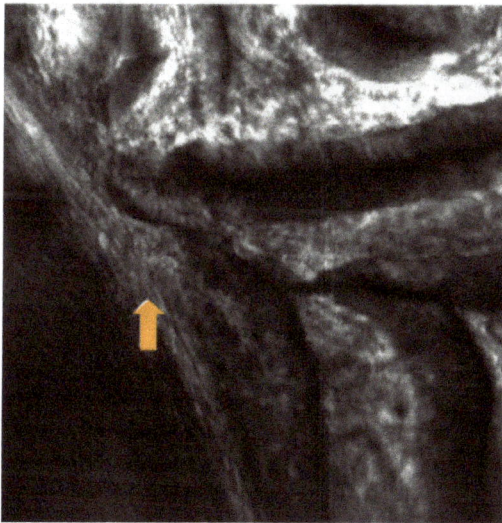

Fig. 3.24. The squamocolumnar junction with the administration of 10% fluorescein sodium. The arrow indicates the junction of squamous epithelium and columnar epithelium. On the columnar epithelial side, the glandular openings are round (deep layer).

References

1. Day DW, Jass JR, Price AB, *et al.* (2003) *Morson and Dawson's Gastrointestinal Pathology*, pp. 21–26.
2. Liu H, Li YQ, Yu T, *et al.* (2009) Confocal laser endomicroscopy for superficial esophageal squamous cell carcinoma. *Endoscopy* **41**: 99–106.

Chapter 4

Gastroesophageal Reflux Disease

Gastroesophageal reflux disease (GERD) is defined as a condition which develops when the reflux of stomach contents causes troublesome symptoms and/or complications according to the Montreal definition.[1] It contains esophageal and extraesophageal syndromes. The esophageal syndromes include the symptomatic syndromes, i.e. the typical reflux syndrome and the reflux chest pain syndrome; and the syndromes with esophageal injury, i.e. reflux esophagitis, reflux stricture, Barrett's esophagus (BE) and esophageal adenocarcinoma.

Esophagogastroduodenoscopy (EGD) is the most frequently requested examination to identify mucosal breaks and to exclude other diseases. Erosive esophagitis is diagnosed by endoscopy when visible breaks are seen in the esophageal mucosa at or immediately above the gastroeophageal junction. Nonerosive reflux disease (NERD) is defined as the presence of troublesome reflux-associated symptoms and the absence of mucosal breaks at endoscopy. Studies have shown that microscopic esophageal mucosal damage has been seen in at least two-thirds of NERD patients. The most commonly seen microscopic features are dilated intercellular space, hyperplasia of the epithelial basal cell, elongation of the intrapapillary capillary loops (IPCLs), and infiltration of inflammatory cells into squamous epithelia. Dilated intercellular space in esophageal epithelium is an extremely sensitive marker of oesophageal damage in GERD, and is also a marker of damage evaluation described for NERD.[2–5]

With its 1000-fold magnifying ability, CLE makes it possible to assess the mucosal layer *in vivo* and enables visualization of the cells of the esophageal squamous epithelium, dilated intercellular space, and IPCLs.

Erosive Reflux Disease

Erosive reflux disease (ERD) can be endoscopically recognized by the presence of mucosal breaks in the esophageal mucosa. Typical presentation under white light endoscopy is erosion or mucosal breaks and the mucosal breaks mixed together along with advancement of inflammation in mucous membrane. According to the Los Angeles (LA) classification system, esophageal erosions were divided into grades A–D.[6]

CLE has been proven to visualize cellular and vascular changes within the esophageal epithelia *in vivo* at high resolution[7] (Fig. 4.1). The dilated intercellular space is an extremely sensitive marker of esophageal epithelia damage in GERD. According to Calabrese, the mean value of the maximum dilated intercellular space in patients with GERD is at least three greater than that in controls.[8] A mean dilated intercellular space of 0.74 μm provides a cutoff score for damage.[2,8] In the Chinese population, intercellular spaces of esophageal epithelial cells in volunteers and erosive esophagitis (EE) patients were 0.37 ± 0.07 μm and 1.33 ± 0.14 μm, respectively[9] (Fig. 4.1C).

IPCLs are readily visible following the intravenous administration of fluorescein sodium (5–10 ml, 10%). More than five IPCLs within the endomicroscopic field of view (500×500 mm) predicted microscopic changes of GERD with a sensitivity of 94.9% (accuracy 91.7%),[7] and elongation of the papillae is often seen in patients with GERD. The elongated IPCLs can reach more than 90% of the total epithelial thickness of the esophgeal membrane in cases of inflammatory reactions and ongoing proliferation (Fig. 4.2). In normal tissue, these papillae are not elongated by more than 10%–20% of the total epithelial thickness.

The other features of ERD by CLE are hyperplasia of the epithelial basal cells and infiltration of inflammatory cells into squamous epithelia, which are difficult to observe due to the limitation on the penetration thickness of CLE.

Nonerosive Reflux Disease

NERD accounts for more than 50% of cases involving GERD,[1,10,11] not only in the West but also in Asia.[12,13] Although patients with NERD

(A)

(B)

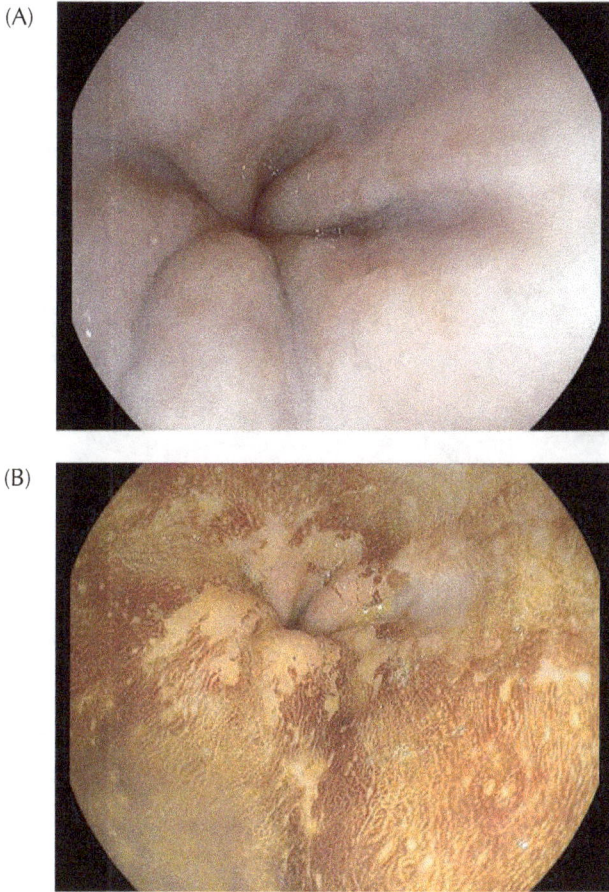

Fig. 4.1. I-scan endoscopic image of the distal oesophagus of erosive reflux disease. The pink–whitish squamous epithelium and mucosal breaks can be easily identified and differentiated from columnar epithelium. (A) Two mucosal breaks no longer than 5 mm, mucosal folds, LA grade A. (B) Mucosal breaks are clearer, owing to sprinkling of Lugol's solution.

have no detectable mucosal breaks at conventional endoscopy, minimal change lesions are often visible upon high-resolution endoscopy in such patients.[14–19] Several studies have employed a modified LA classification system, in which two grades, grade N (esophagus without any mucosal breaks or minimal changes) and grade M (minimal changes

(A)

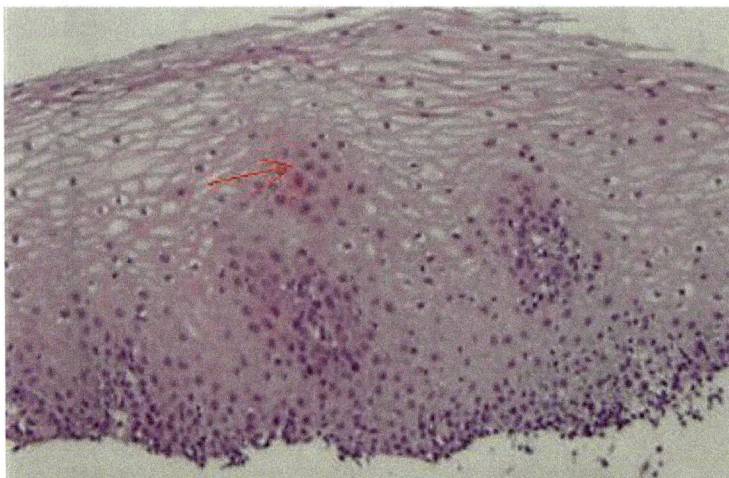

(B)

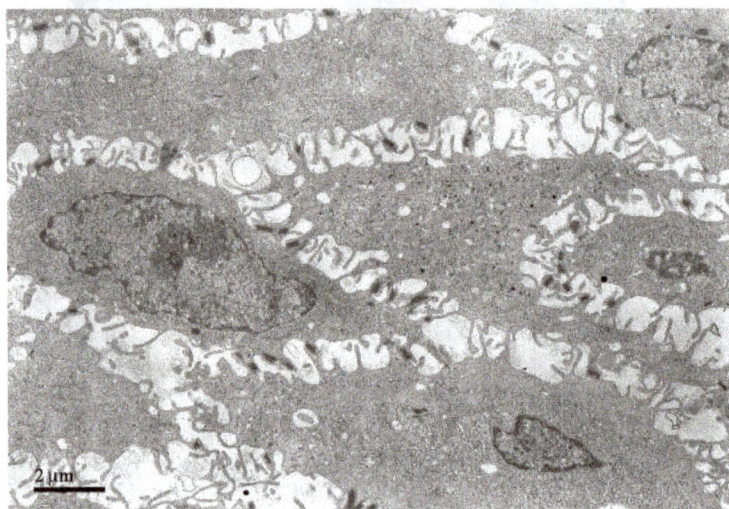

Fig. 4.2.   Endomicroscopy of erosive reflux disease. (A) Conventional histology of the squamous epithelium. Dilatation of intercellular spaces is visible. The basal layer is increased in thickness (*arrow*). IPCLs are elongated, reaching more than 70% of the total epithelial thickness of the esophageal membrane (HE × 400). (B) Transmission electron microscopy image showing the dilated intercellular spaces (original magnification × 7000; scale bar = 2 μm). (C) Endomicroscopic image of surface squamous epithelium of ERD. Marked dilatation of intercellular spaces and an increased number of IPCLs are visible (*arrow*); the boundary of the prickle cell is obscured. (D) Intrapapillary loops (*arrow*) and squamous epithelium in the deeper portion of the mucosa.

(C)

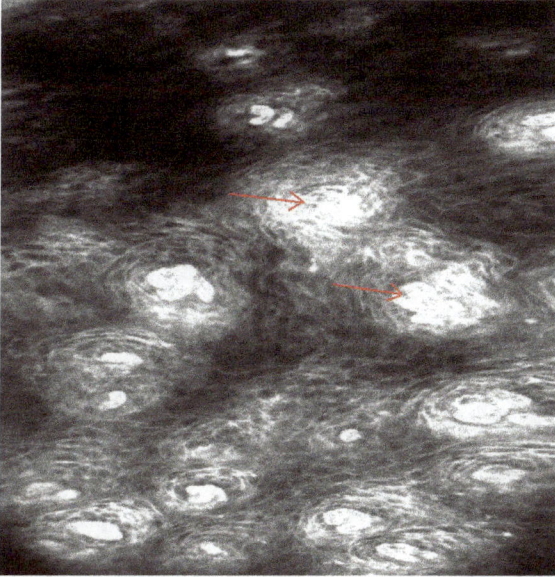

(D)

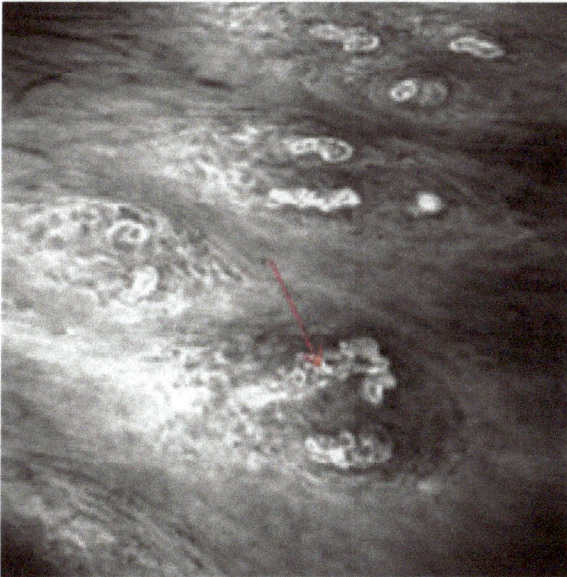

Fig. 4.2. (*Continued*)

(A)

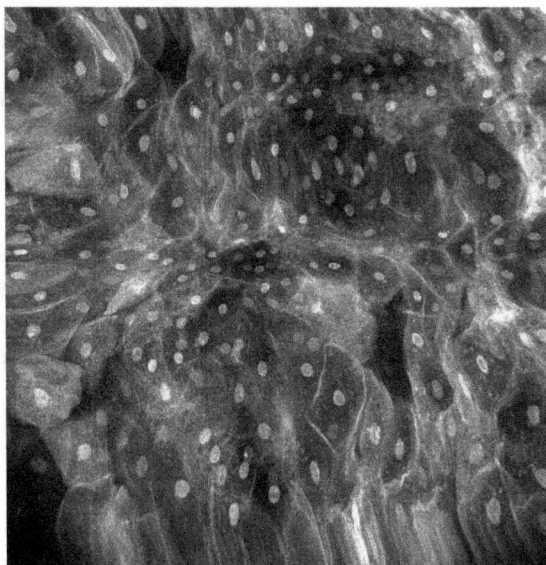

(B)

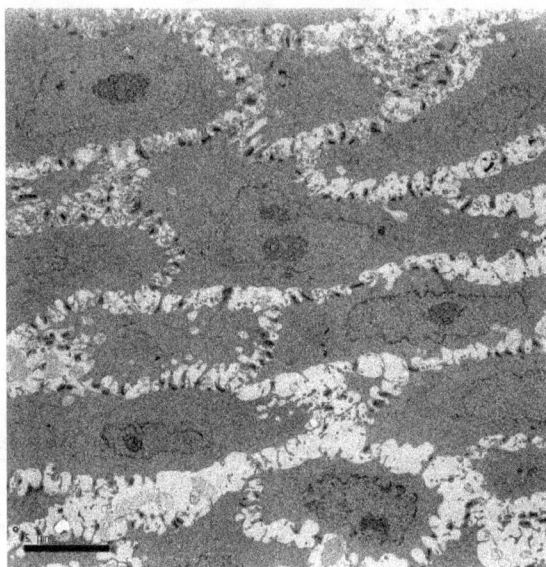

Fig. 4.3.   Nonerosive reflux disease: I-scan endoscopic image of NERD. (A) Endomicroscopic image of the surface layer squamous epithelium with visible nuclei (arrow) after acriflavine staining. IPCLs have prolonged to the surface squamous epithelium layer. (B) Corresponding transmission electron image with dilated intercellular spaces (original magnification × 7000; scale bar = 2 μm)

(C)

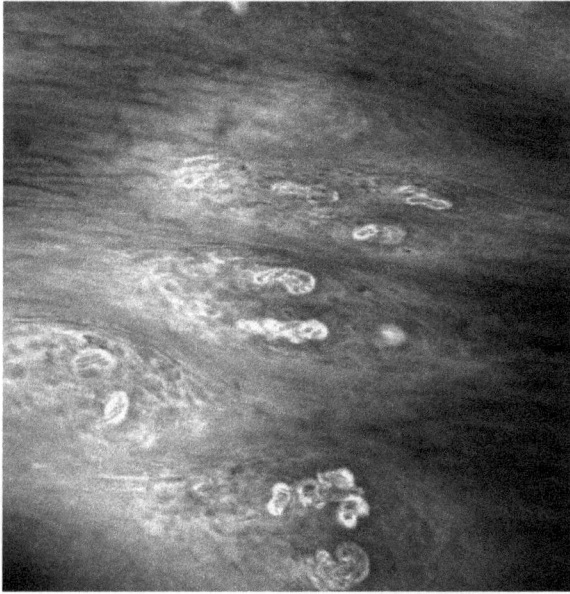

Fig. 4.3. (*Continued*) (C) Elongated IPCLs and dilated intercellular spaces in the middle depth of the squamous epithelium.

such as erythema without sharp demarcation, whitish turbidity, and/or invisibility of vessels), are added to the usual LA grades, A–D.[6,17,18]

As with ERD, dilated intercellular spaces and an increased number of elongated IPCLs are the most common features in patients with NERD by CLE.[4,20] The nuclei of squamous epithelium can be easily stained and the dilated intercellular space would be clearer with acriflavine (concentration of 0.02%) sprinkled (Fig. 4.3).

References

1. Vakil N, van Zanten SV, Kahrilas P, *et al.* (2006) The Montreal definition and classification of gastroesophageal reflux disease: a global evidence-based consensus. *Am J Gastroenterol* **101**: 1900–1920; quiz 1943.

2. Orlando LA, Orlando RC. (2009) Dilated intercellular spaces as a marker of GERD. *Curr Gastroenterol Rep* **11**: 190–194.

3. van Malenstein H, Farre R, Sifrim D. (2008) Esophageal dilated inter-cellular spaces (DIS) and nonerosive reflux disease. *Am J Gastroenterol* **103**: 1021–1028.

4. Caviglia R, Ribolsi M, Maggiano N, *et al.* (2005) Dilated intercellular spaces of esophageal epithelium in nonerosive reflux disease patients with physiological esophageal acid exposure. *Am J Gastroenterol* **100**: 543–548.

5. Farre R, De Vos R, Geboes K, *et al.* (2007) Critical role of stress in increased oesophageal mucosa permeability and dilated intercellular spaces. *Gut* **56**: 1191–1197.

6. Lundell LR, Dent J, Bennett JR, *et al.* (1999) Endoscopic assessment of oesophagitis: clinical and functional correlates and further validation of the Los Angeles classification. *Gut* **45**: 172–180.

7. Kiesslich R, Lammersdorf K, Goetz M, *et al.* (2006) Microscopic changes in non-erosive reflux disease (NERD) can be diagnosed during ongoing endoscopy by confocal laser endomicroscopy (CLE). *Gastrointest Endosc* **63**: AB243–AB243.

8. Calabrese C, Fabbri A, Bortolotti M, *et al.* (2003) Dilated intercellular spaces as a marker of oesophageal damage: comparative results in gastro-oesophageal reflux disease with or without bile reflux. *Aliment Pharmacol Ther* **18**: 525–532.

9. Xue Y, Zhou LY, Lin SR. (2008) Dilated intercellular spaces in gastroe-sophageal reflux disease patients and the changes of intercellular spaces after omeprazole treatment. *Chin Med J (Engl)* **121**: 1297–1301.

10. Mishima I, Adachi K, Arima N, *et al.* (2005) Prevalence of endoscopically negative and positive gastroesophageal reflux disease in the Japanese. *Scand J Gastroenterol* **40**: 1005–1009.

11. Fass R. (2007) Erosive esophagitis and nonerosive reflux disease (NERD): comparison of epidemiologic, physiologic, and therapeutic characteristics. *J Clin Gastroenterol* **41**: 131–137.

12. Dent J, El-Serag HB, Wallander MA, Johansson S. (2005) Epidemiology of gastro-oesophageal reflux disease: a systematic review. *Gut* **54**: 710–717.

13. Wong BC, Kinoshita Y. (2006) Systematic review on epidemiology of gastroesophageal reflux disease in Asia. *Clin Gastroenterol Hepatol* **4**: 398–407.

14. Sharma P, Wani S, Bansal A, *et al.* (2007) A feasibility trial of narrow band imaging endoscopy in patients with gastroesophageal reflux disease. *Gastroenterology* **133**: 454–464; quiz 674.
15. Gossner L. (2008) Potential contribution of novel imaging modalities in non-erosive reflux disease. *Best Pract Res Clin Gastroenterol* **22**: 617–624.
16. Kiesslich R, Kanzler S, Vieth M, *et al.* (2004) Minimal change esophagitis: prospective comparison of endoscopic and histological markers between patients with non-erosive reflux disease and normal controls using magnifying endoscopy. *Dig Dis* **22**: 221–227.
17. Lee JH, Kim N, Chung IK, *et al.* (2008) Clinical significance of minimal change lesions of the esophagus in a healthy Korean population: a nationwide multi-center prospective study. *J Gastroenterol Hepatol* **23**: 1153–1157.
18. Kusano M, Shirai N, Yamaguchi K, *et al.* (2008) It is possible to classify non-erosive reflux disease (NERD) patients into endoscopically normal groups and minimal change groups by subjective symptoms and responsiveness to rabeprazole — a report from a study with Japanese patients. *Dig Dis Sci* **53**: 3082–3094.
19. Nakamura T, Shirakawa K, Masuyama H, *et al.* (2005) Minimal change oesophagitis: a disease with characteristic differences to erosive oesophagitis. *Aliment Pharmacol Ther* **21** (Suppl 2): 19–26.
20. Caviglia R, Ribolsi M, Gentile M, *et al.* (2007) Dilated intercellular spaces and acid reflux at the distal and proximal oesophagus in patients with non-erosive gastro-oesophageal reflux disease. *Aliment Pharmacol Ther* **25**: 629–636.

Chapter 5

Barrett's Esophagus and Esophageal Adenocarcinoma

Barrett's Esophagus

Barrett's esophagus (BE) is defined as a pathological change from the normal stratified squamous epithelium of the lower esophagus to a metaplastic columnar epithelium.[1] It is widely recognized as a premalignant condition of esophageal adenocarcinoma, a tumor with an increasing incidence in most Western countries.[2] BE is found in 1.6% of the general population and in 10% of those patients undergoing endoscopy for gastroesophageal reflux symptoms.[3]

BE can be endoscopically identified by its velvety red mucosa (compared with the normal, pale esophageal mucosa) over the gastroesophageal junction (GEJ). The extending columnar epithelium in the lower esophagus can have either a circumferential or tongue-like appearance, or a combination of these two patterns (Figs. 5.1 and 3.4). It was initially considered that the columnar mucosa had to extend by at least on 3 cm over the GEJ in order to diagnose BE. But this definition has changed, due to the recognition of short segment BE measuring less than 3 cm. Another newly developed endoscopic standardization of BE is the Prague classification system of circumferential (C) and maximal length (M). This classification distinguishes the landmarks of the squamocolumnar junction, the GEJ, the extent of the circumferential columnar lining, and the maximal columnar extension excluding islands to determine the length of BE. However, columnar islands and ultrashort BE <1 cm are not included in this system.

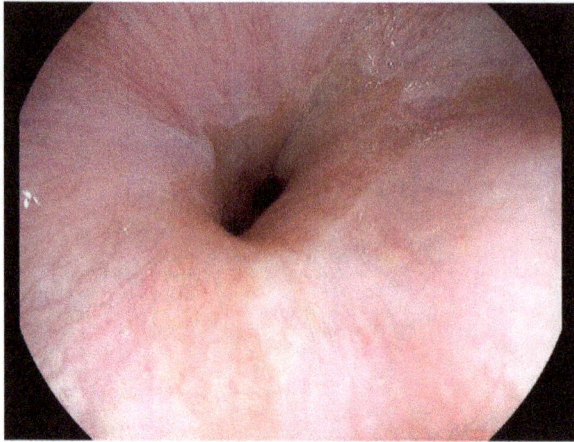

Fig. 5.1.   White-light endoscopic view of the distal esophagus, showing a short, tongue-like, reddish columnar mucosa.

The diagnosis of BE is based on both endoscopy and histology. Three distinct types of epithelium can be present in BE: oxyntic type epithelium (parietal and chief cells are present), and cardiac and intestinal type epithelium (also called specialized intestinal metaplasia (IM) or junctional type epithelium). However, there is at present a controversy over whether the presence of IM is a prerequisite for the diagnosis of BE. The diagnostic criteria proposed by various societies and groups are summarized in Table 5.1.

IM of the esophagus, similar to type II and type III IM of the stomach, is considered as an incomplete form of IM. The epithelium of Barrett's intestinal mucosa is composed mainly of goblet cells interspersed among intermediate mucous cells (Fig. 5.10). It is rare to detect mature absorptive intestinal cells with a well-defined brush border in BE. Except in children, IM is the most common type in Barrett's epithelium. Viewing from the standpoint of the risk of developing adenocarcinoma, only a columnar lined esophagus with IM has malignant potential. The length of the columnar segment is the strongest predictor of Barrett's IM at endoscopy.[4] However, various histological patterns cannot be distinguished under standard endoscopy. Since IM is patchy in distribution, multiple biopsies are

Table 5.1. Diagnostic Criteria for Barrett's Esophagus Proposed by Various Societies[9]

	Endoscopy Shows Columnar-lined Lower Esophagus	Biopsy Specimens Show Intestinal Metaplasia
AGA–ACG	Yes	Yes
GSP	Yes	Yes
Amsterdam IG	Yes	Yes
Montreal IG	Yes	Or gastric metaplasia
BSG	Yes	No

AGA — American Gastroenterological Association; ACG — American College of Gastroenterology; GSP — German Society of Pathology; IG — International Group; BSG — British Society of Gastroenterology.

required to make this diagnosis. The Seattle protocol recommended a biopsy protocol with four-quadrant biopsies every 1 cm (in short segment BE) or 2 cm (in long segment BE). However, considering the greatly increased examination time for the endoscopist and the workload for the histopathologist, this biopsy protocol is hard to complete for most gastroenterologists in clinical practice.

CLE enables subsurface imaging of the columnar lined mucosa during ongoing endoscopy, and can easily identify goblet cells in the metaplastic epithelium. The first study to apply CLE for the diagnosis of BE was reported in 2006, and the confocal Barrett classification was established based on a comparison of the *in vivo* and conventional *ex vivo* histology (Table 5.2).[5] Following retrospective comparison between the 3012 confocal images obtained from 156 areas and corresponding histopathological results showed that BE could be predicted by CLE with a sensitivity of 98.1% and a specificity of 94.1%. In addition, this classification could diagnose Barrett's-associated neoplastic changes with a sensitivity of 92.9% and a specificity of 98.4%, respectively.

Endomicroscopic imaging of Barrett's epithelium is similar to that of corresponding histopathological features. The fundic and cardiac type Barrett's epithelium shows regular-shaped glands with round or oval openings (Figs. 5.2 and 5.5). The columnar epithelium preserves good polarity and regular arrangement. For Barrett's glands with

Table 5.2.   Endomicroscopic Classification of Barrett's Esophagus[5]

Confocal Diagnosis	Vessel Architecture	Crypt Architecture
Gastric type epithelium	Capillaries with a regular shape, visible only in the deeper parts of the mucosal layer.	Regular columnar-lined epithelium with round glandular openings and typical cobblestone appearance.
Barrett's epithelium	Subepithelial capillaries with a regular shape underneath columnar-lined epithelium, visible in the upper and deeper parts of the mucosal layer.	Columnar lined epithelium with intermittent dark mucin in goblet cells in the upper parts of the mucosal layer. In the deeper parts, villous, dark, regular cylindrical Barrett's epithelial cells are present.
Neoplasia	Irregular capillaries, visible in the upper and deeper parts of the mucosal layer. Leakage of vessels leads to a heterogeneous and brighter signal intensity within the lamina propria.	Black cells with irregular apical and distal borders and shapes, with strong dark contrast against the surrounding tissue.

specialized IM (typical Barrett's epithelium), goblet cells can be observed interspersed between columnar epithelium (Figs. 5.8 and 5.9). High grade intraepithelial neoplasia and early esophageal adenocarcinoma can be recognized by a characteristic glandular and cell type in CLE imaging. The heterogeneous-shaped glands are mainly composed of irregular and elongated epithelial cells (Fig. 5.12).

Later, a randomized, crossover study was conducted prospectively to compare the diagnostic yield between standard endoscopy with random biopsy and endomicroscopy with targeted biopsy.[6] The results revealed that CLE with targeted biopsy improved the diagnostic yield for the detection of endoscopically inapparent Barrett's neoplasia from 17% to 33%. In patients undergoing surveillance endoscopy for BE, almost two-thirds did not need any biopsy at all, because no neoplasia

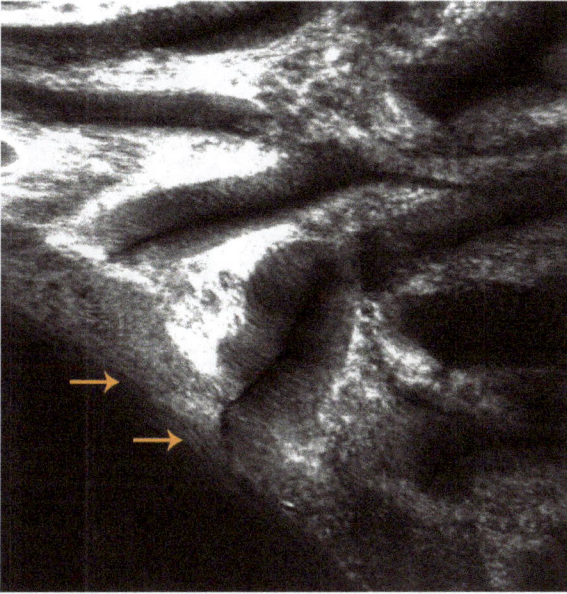

Fig. 5.2. The endomicroscopic image of this area shows regularly arranged glands with enlarged openings, indicating a cardiac type epithelium of Barrett's mucosa; cylindrical columnar epithelial cells with good polarity; homogeneous distributed fluorescein in the interstitium, showing highlighting bright regions; and the squamo-columnar junction (*arrows*) is distinct with the lower left squamous epithelium and upper right columnar epithelium.

was detected during endomicroscopic imaging. Thus, CLE can allow immediate and reliable diagnosis of BE and Barrett's-associated neoplasia during endoscopic examination with less biopsy to be performed. Furthermore, a case report has shown the application of CLE in targeted EMR of focal high grade intraepithelial neoplasia.[7]

Adenocarcinoma

The incidence of esophageal adenocarcinoma has been rising since the mid-1970s, and in 1994 the number of patients with adenocarcinoma of the esophagus exceeded that of patients with squamous cell carcinoma. A large majority of adenocarcinomas of the esophagus have arisen from BE.

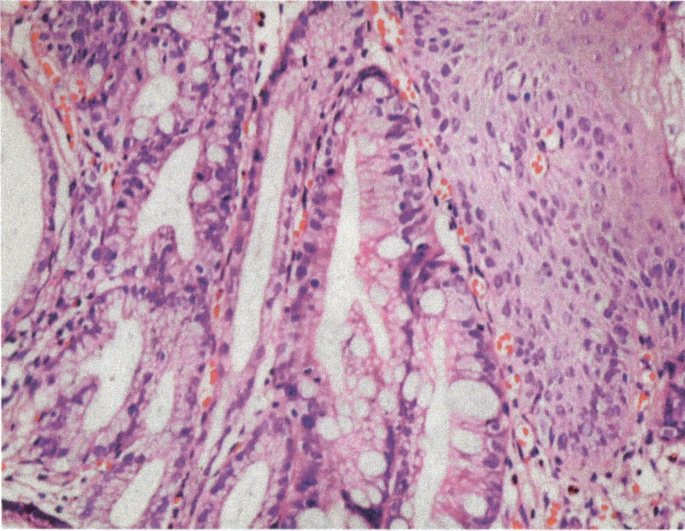

Fig. 5.3.   The corresponding histopathology shows Barrett's esophagus with cardiac type epithelium.

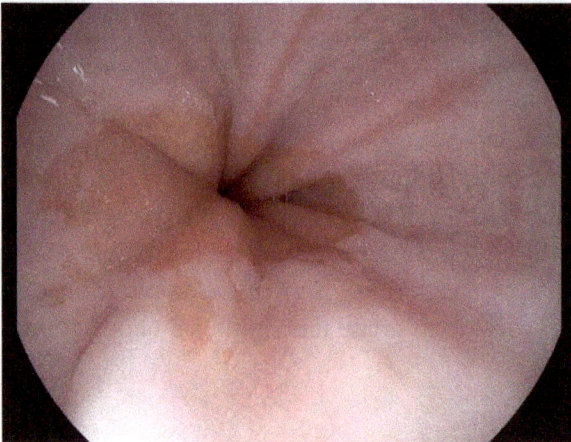

Fig. 5.4.   White-light endoscopy shows a semicircular reddish mucosa with several irregular mucosal islands in the distal esophagus.

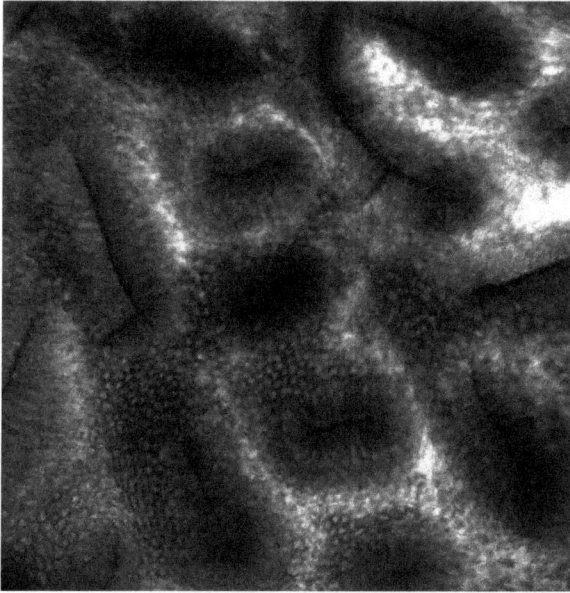

Fig. 5.5. Endomicroscopy displays regular-shaped columnar epithelial cells within the distal esophagus, suggesting Barrett's epithelium; the glands show a mixed pattern, with both the cardiac type (enlarged openings) and the oxyntic type epithelium presented.

Similar to adenocarcinomas arising in the stomach, the majority of esophageal adenocarcinomas have a tubular or papillary pattern of the intestinal type.[8] Most adenocarcinomas are advanced at the time of endoscopic examination, with obvious intramural and adventitial involvement. Considering the technical difficulty in performing biopsy at the GEJ and massive bleeding caused by multiple sampling, false negative histological diagnosis does exist in many cases. However, distinct characteristics of the cancerous tissue can be observed in endomicroscopic images, such as disorganized or even disappeared glandular structure, black malignant cells with irregular shape, loss of a regular basal border, and heterogeneous brightness of the interstitium due to neoangiogenesis and fluorescein leakage (Figs. 5.15, 5.16 and 5.19). Therefore, under the guide of endomicroscopic imaging, targeted biopsies can provide more accurate sampling of the macroscopic lesions and highly improve the histological detection rate of esophageal adenocarcima.

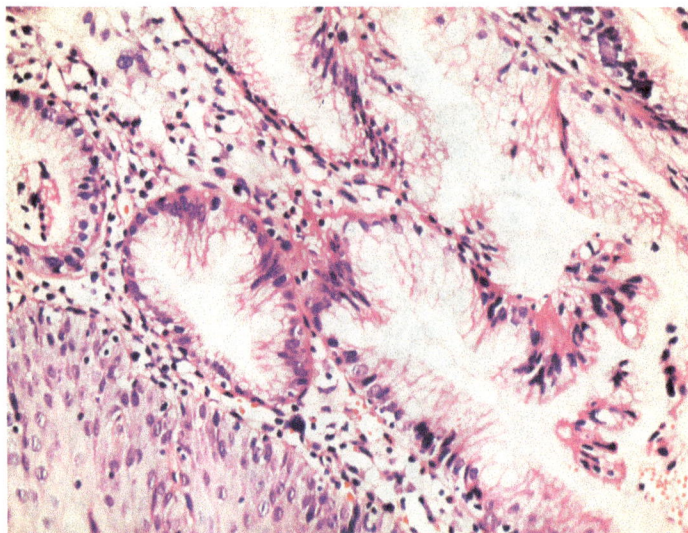

Fig. 5.6. Histopathology of the targeted biopsy shows Barrett's epithelium with cardiac type and oxyntic type epithelium.

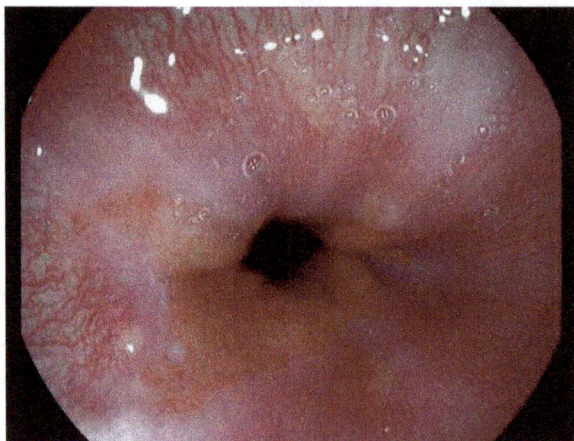

Fig. 5.7. Several irregular-shaped reddish mucosas were observed in the distal esophagus.

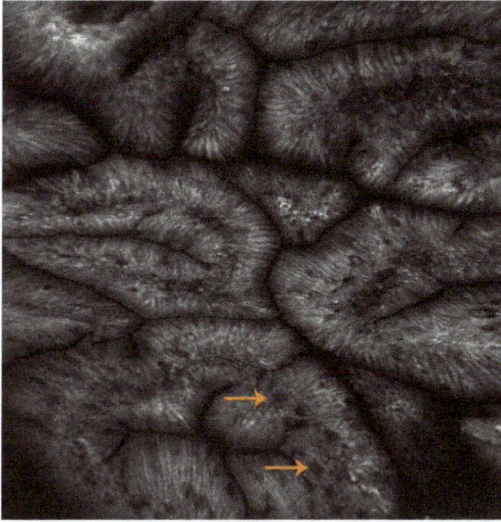

Fig. 5.8. In the upper parts of the mucosal layer of Barrett's epithelium, endomicroscopy shows typical villiform epithelium. Goblet cells with dark mucin (*arrows*) are present within the columnar epithelium, suggesting intestinal type Barrett's mucosa.

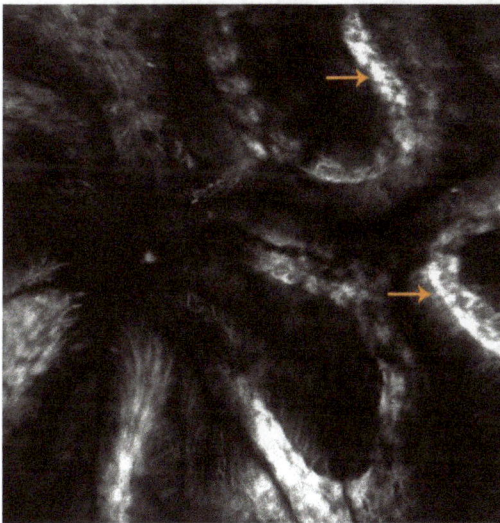

Fig. 5.9. The deeper parts of the mucosal layer of Barrett's epithelium are displayed as a homogeneous dark band with clear apical and basal borders. The subepithelial capillaries (*arrows*) are easily recognizable and regular in shape.

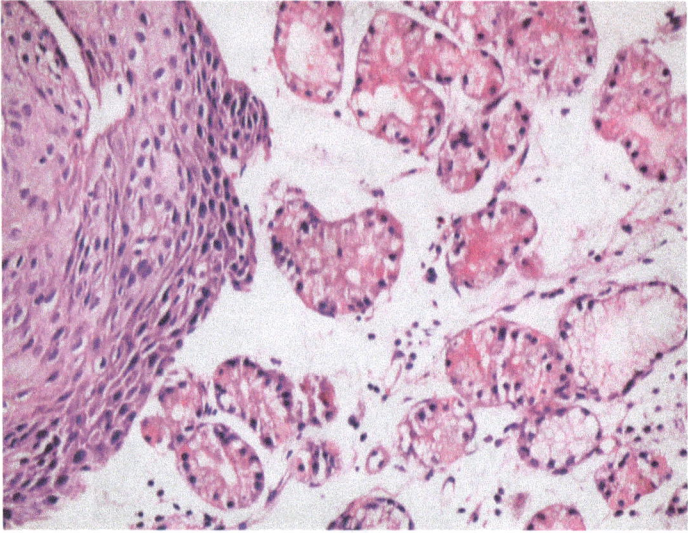

Fig. 5.10.   The corresponding histopathology of the CLE-examined mucosa shows intestinal type Barrett's epithelium.

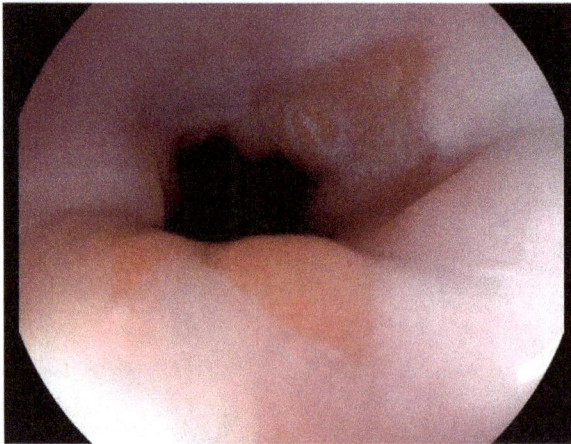

Fig. 5.11.   A shallow elevated lesion is visible within the distal esophagus in white-light endoscopy.

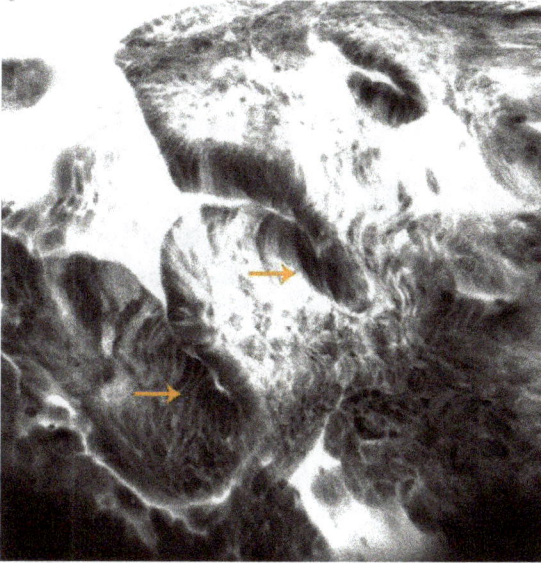

Fig. 5.12.   Endomicroscopy of this lesion shows distorted, irregular-shaped glands (*arrows*) with dark irregular epithelial cells. Heterogeneous fluorescein leakage is visible due to angiogenesis of the local mucosa.

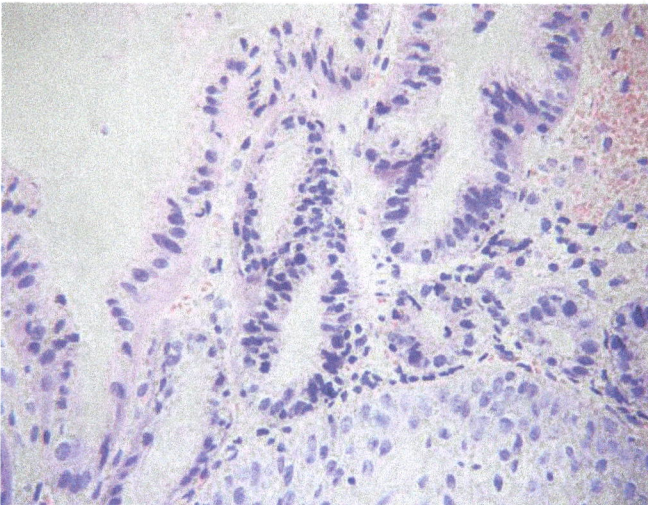

Fig. 5.13.   Histopathology confirmed Barrett's esophagus with intraepithelial neoplasia.

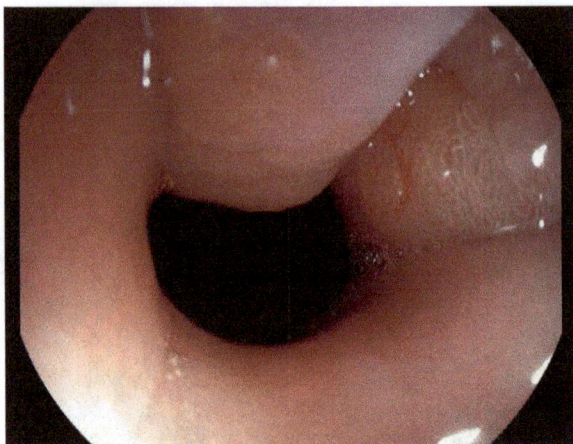

Fig. 5.14.   White-light endoscopic image of the distal esophagus, showing a superficial protrusion and mild bleeding.

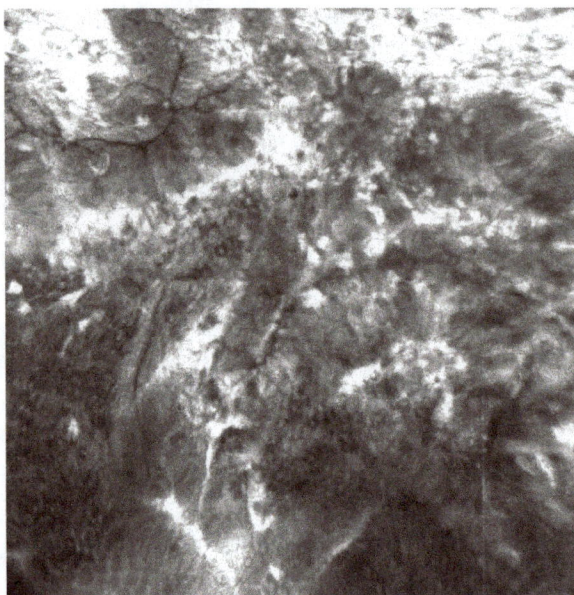

Fig. 5.15.   The gland architecture becomes highly irregular and deranged, with loss of polarity of the epithelial cells. Strong leakage of the epithelial capillaries is observed with pooling of fluorescein in the lamina propria, suggesting neoangiogenesis.

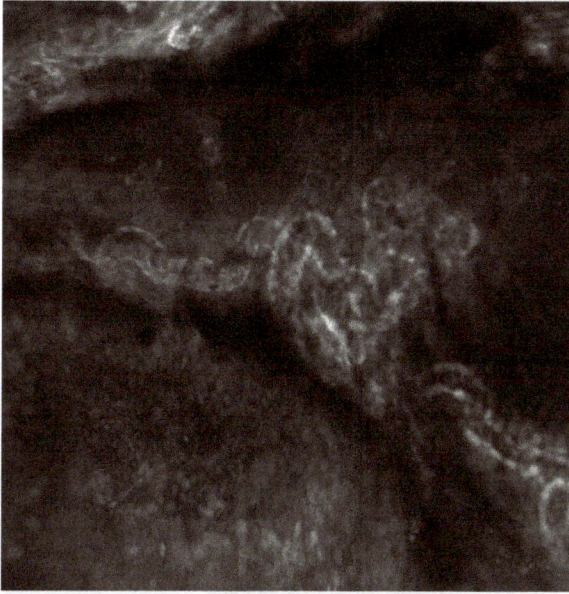

Fig. 5.16. In the deeper part of the disrupted mucosa, endomicroscopy displays severely distorted subepithelial capillaries with an increased caliber.

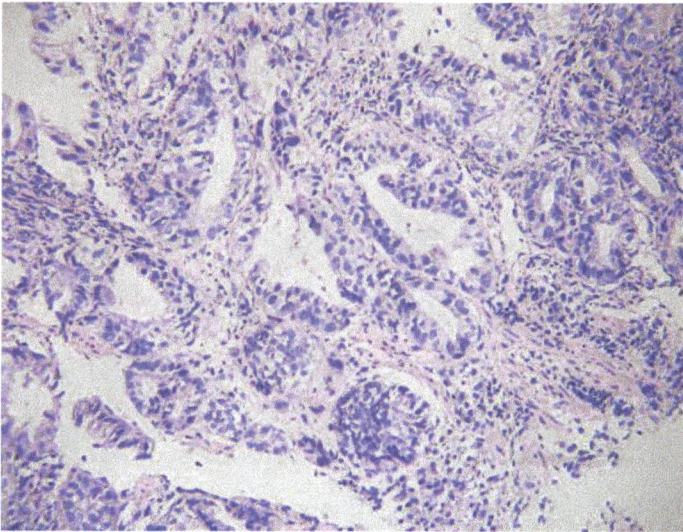

Fig. 5.17. The corresponding histopathology confirms well-differentiated adeno-carcinoma of the esophagus.

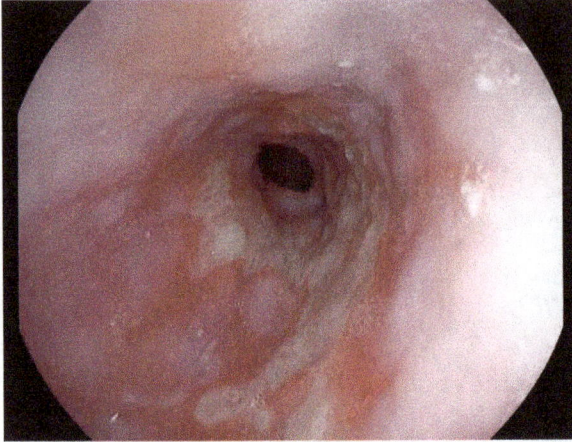

Fig. 5.18.   White-light endoscopy of the distal esophagus shows circumferential erosion with surface unevenness.

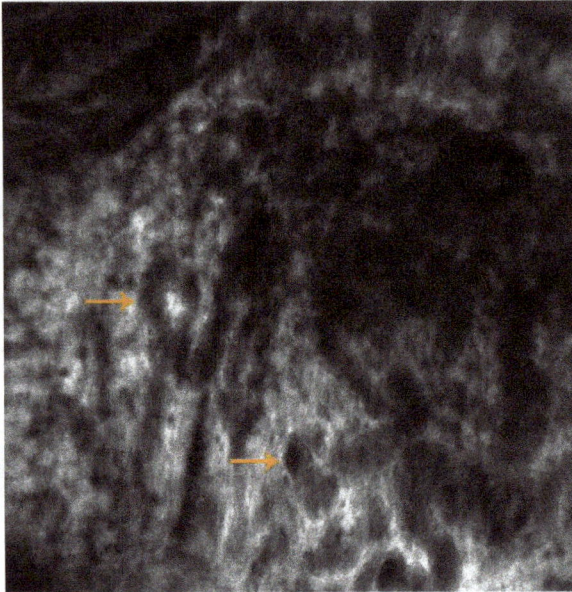

Fig. 5.19.   Endomicroscopy displays the overall loss of normal crypt architecture, with only several severely altered glandular structures (*arrows*), and the cell polarity is completely disturbed.

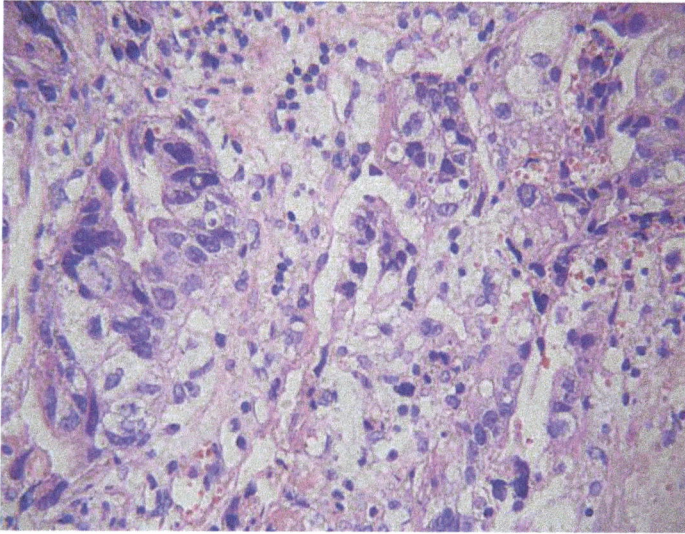

Fig. 5.20. Histopathology shows undifferentiated esophageal adenocarcinoma.

References

1. Spechler SJ, Goyal RK. (1996) The columnar-lined esophagus, intestinal metaplasia, and Norman Barrett. *Gastroenterology* **110**: 614–621.
2. Haggitt RC. (1992) Adenocarcinoma in Barrett's esophagus: a new epidemic? *Hum Pathol* **23**: 475–476.
3. Ronkainen J, Aro P, Storskrubb T, *et al.* (2005) Prevalence of Barrett's esophagus in the general population: an endoscopic study. *Gastroenterology* **129**: 1825–1831.
4. Jego M, Volant A, Faycal J, *et al.* (2007) Prevalence and topography of intestinal metaplasia in columnar lined esophagus. *Gastroenterol Clin Biol* **31**: 601–606.
5. Kiesslich R, Gossner L, Goetz M, *et al.* (2006) *In vivo* histology of Barrett's esophagus and associated neoplasia by confocal laser endomicroscopy. *Clin Gastroenterol Hepatol* **4**: 979–987.
6. Dunbar KB, Okolo P, 3rd, Montgomery E, Canto MI. (2009) Confocal laser endomicroscopy in Barrett's esophagus and endoscopically inapparent Barrett's neoplasia: a prospective, randomized, double-blind, controlled, crossover trial. *Gastrointest Endosc* **70**: 645–654.

7. Leung KK, Maru D, Abraham S, *et al.* (2009) Optical EMR: confocal endomicroscopy-targeted EMR of focal high-grade dysplasia in Barrett's esophagus. *Gastrointest Endosc* **69**: 170–172.

8. Lauren P. (1965) The two histological main types of gastric carcinoma: diffuse and so-called intestinal-type carcinoma. An attempt at a histo-clinical classification. *Acta Pathol Microbiol Scand* **64**: 31–49.

9. Flejou JF. (2008) Histological assessment of oesophageal columnar mucosa. *Best Pract Res Clin Gastroenterol* **22**: 671–686.

Chapter 6

Esophageal Squamous Cell Carcinoma

Although relatively infrequent in Western countries, esophageal squamous cell carcinoma (SCC) is still a major disease for a large proportion of the world's population, especially in China and Japan.[1,2] The prognosis for SCC is poor because it is usually diagnosed at an advanced stage. Early detection is still regarded as the best option for improving the prognosis of this disease, and endoscopy is one of the most widely used techniques for early diagnosis. However, early SCC is frequently multifocal and hard to detect by conventional endoscopy. Endoscopic appearances include flat lesions with color variation, focal red areas, nodules, or erosions (Fig. 6.1). It has been

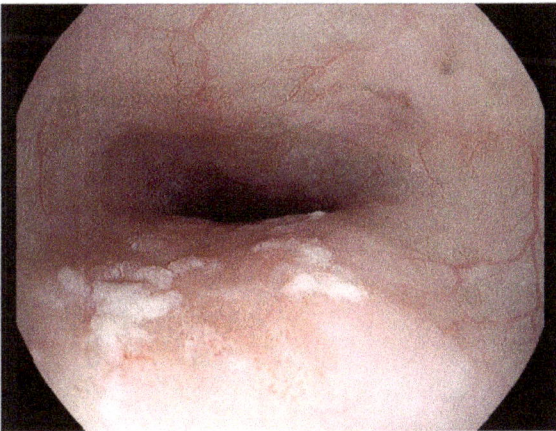

Fig. 6.1. Endoscopic appearance of superficial esophageal squamous cell carcinoma.

reported that iodine staining, magnifying endoscopy, and narrow band imaging can improve the early diagnosis of esophageal cancer by providing details of the esophageal surface (Figs. 6.2 and 6.3).[3–5] Both endocytoscopy and CLE have enabled examination of cellular

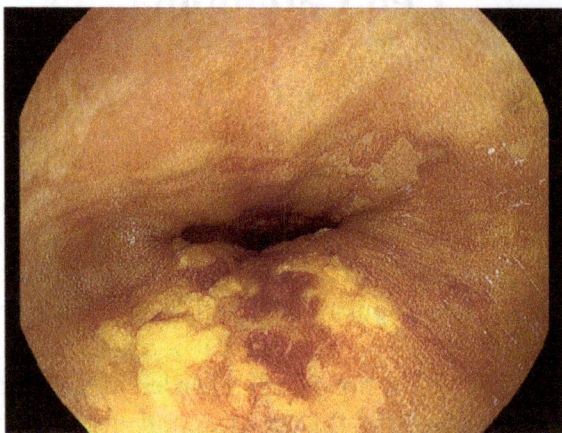

Fig. 6.2. Endoscopic appearance of superficial esophageal squamous cell carcinoma, with iodine staining.

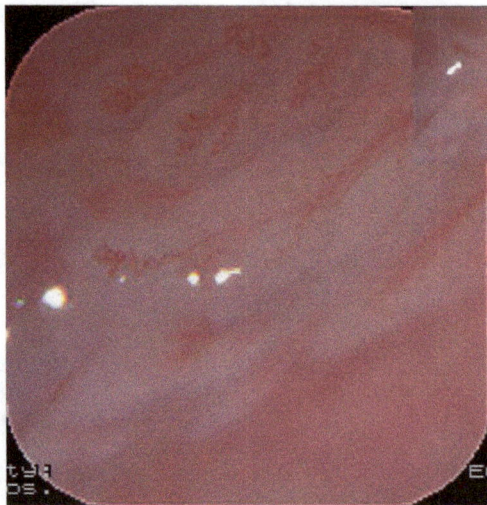

Fig. 6.3. Magnified endoscopic image of superficial esophageal squamous cell carcinoma. Long branching IPCLs and increased diameter of IPCLs are observed.

changes during ongoing endoscopy; CLE allows observation of not only squamous epithelial cells but also the vascular networks of the mucosal layer.[6,7]

Morphological features of squamous cell dysplasia and carcinoma include both architectural and cytological abnormalities.[8] Irregularly arranged squamous epithelial cells, increased diameter of IPCLs, massive IPCLs with tortuous appearance, and long branching IPCLs were effective features in diagnosing SCC.

The CLE images of SCC showed darker esophageal squamous cells with irregular and heterogeneous arrangement; the cellular border is obscured. The nucleus could not easily be identified due to the use of fluorescein sodium as the contrast agent (Fig. 6.4). Topical acriflavine can improve the sensitivity and specificity. Furthermore, it allows better differentiation between intraepithelial neoplasia and cancer by using the shape and arrangement of cells. The nuclei within the epithelium appear denser in SCC, and the cytological abnormality is

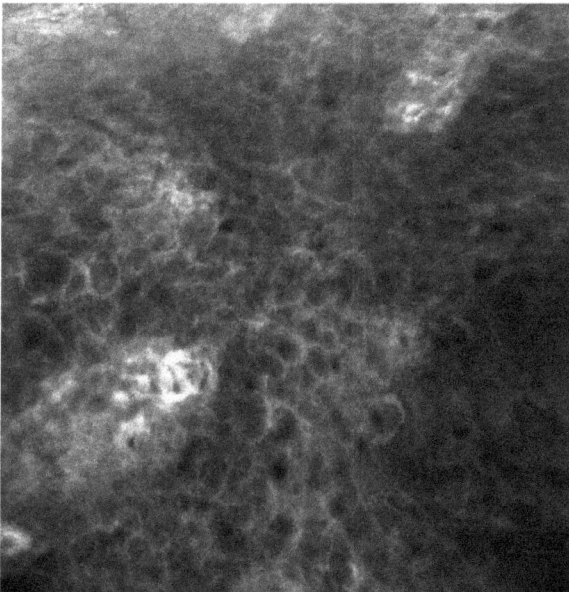

Fig. 6.4. Endomicroscopic characteristics of esophageal squamous epithelial cells. Heterogeneous and darker squamous epithelial cells with irregular arrangement.

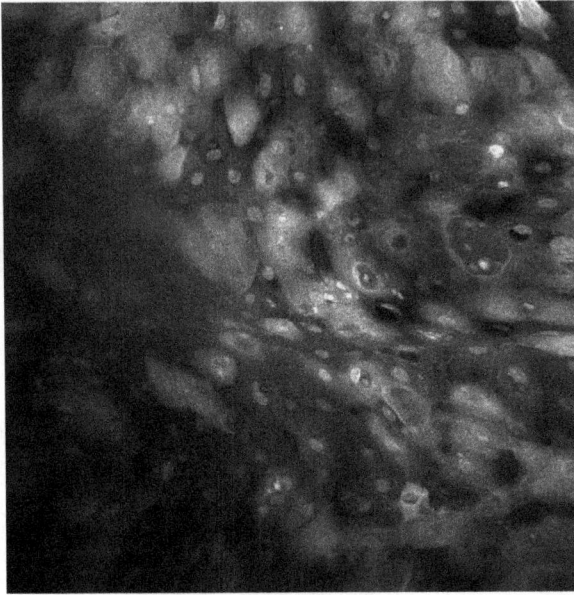

Fig. 6.5.   The nuclei are visible after topical application of acriflavine. The cytological abnormality is characterized by nuclear pleomorphism; the nuclear/cytoplasmic ratio is increased.

characterized by nuclear enlargement, hyperchromasia, and an increased nuclear/cytoplasmic ratio (Fig. 6.5).

IPCLs are the distinct microvascular characteristic of esophageal epithelium. The number, caliber, and shape of IPCLs were changed in cancerous epithelium (Figs. 6.6 and 6.7), and capillary leakage was frequently present (Fig. 6.1).

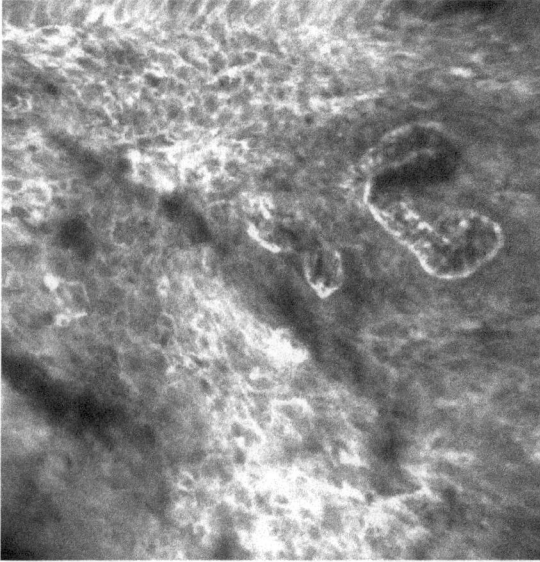

Fig. 6.6. IPCLs with an increased diameter.

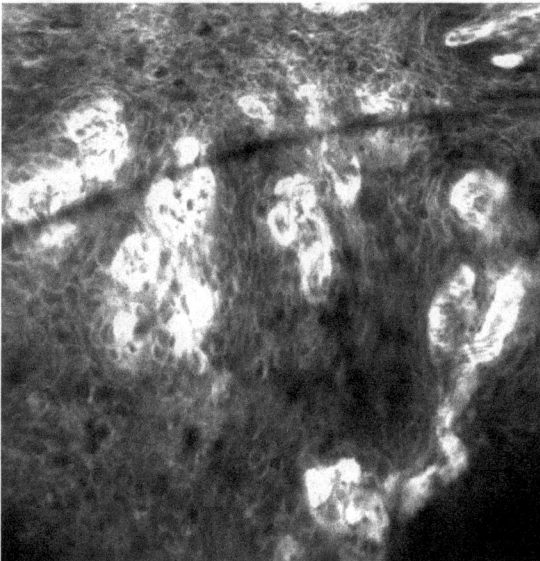

Fig. 6.7. Massive IPCLs with tortuous vessels and long branching IPCLs.

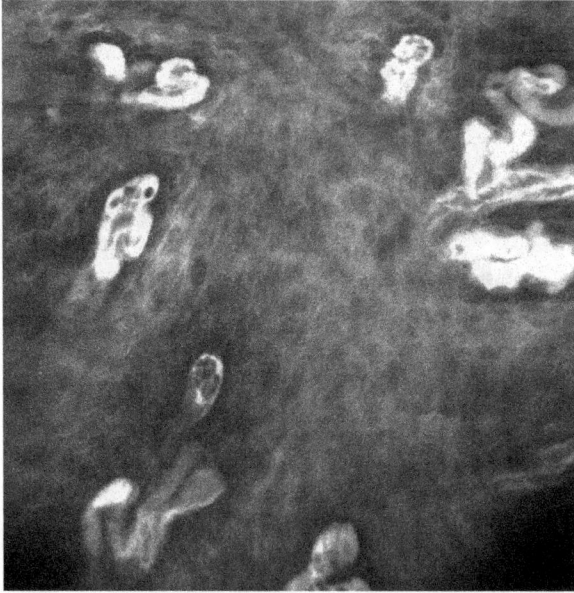

Fig. 6.8.   IPCLs of different sizes, distributed unevenly.

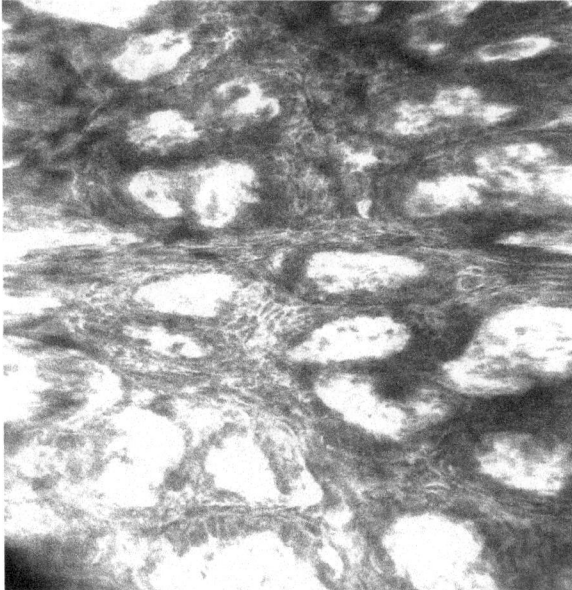

Fig. 6.9.   The margins of IPCLs are sometimes obscured, with capillary leakage.

References

1. Messmann H. (2001) Squamous cell cancer of the oesophagus. *Best Pract Res Clin Gastroenterol* **15**: 249–265.
2. Wang GQ, Abnet CC, Shen Q, *et al.* (2005) Histological precursors of oesophageal squamous cell carcinoma: results from a 13-year prospective follow-up study in a high risk population. *Gut* **54**: 187–192.
3. Inoue H, Rey JF, Lightdale C. (2001) Lugol chromoendoscopy for esophageal squamous cell cancer. *Endoscopy* **33**: 75–79.
4. Kara MA, Peters FP, Fockens P, *et al.* (2006) Endoscopic video-autofluorescence imaging followed by narrow band imaging for detecting early neoplasia in Barrett's esophagus. *Gastrointest Endosc* **64**: 176–185.
5. Sasajima K, Kudo SE, Inoue H, *et al.* (2006) Real-time *in vivo* virtual histology of colorectal lesions when using the endocytoscopy system. *Gastrointest Endosc* **63**: 1010–1017.
6. Liu H, Li YQ, Yu T, *et al.* (2009) Confocal laser endomicroscopy for superficial esophageal squamous cell carcinoma. *Endoscopy* **41**: 99–106.
7. Pech O, Rabenstein T, Manner H, *et al.* (2008) Confocal laser endomicroscopy for *in vivo* diagnosis of early squamous cell carcinoma in the esophagus. *Clin Gastroenterol Hepatol* **6**: 89–94.
8. Takubo K, Aida J, Sawabe M, *et al.* (2007) Early squamous cell carcinoma of the oesophagus: the Japanese viewpoint. *Histopathology* **51**: 733–742.
9. Gabbert HE, Shimoda T, Hainaut P, *et al.* (2000) Squamous cell carcinoma of the oesophagus. In: Hamilton SR, Aaltonen LH (eds.), *Pathology and Genetics of Tumours of the Digestive System: World Health Organization Classification of Tumours*. IARC, Lyon, pp. 11–19.

Chapter 7

Miscellaneous Diseases of the Esophagus

Heterotopic Gastric Mucosa in the Esophagus

Generally speaking, columnar mucosa can be present among the squamous epithelium of the esophagus under two conditions: Barrett's esophagus and heterotopic gastric mucosa (HGM). In fact, HGM is not exclusively found in the esophagus, as it is also present in the tongue, duodenum, jejunum, gall bladder, and rectum.[1-4] The incidence of HGM in the esophagus varies from 5% to 10% in Western countries and 0.1% to 1% in China. Esophageal HGM is generally regarded as a congenital condition, and is frequent in the cervical esophagus. Most of its carriers are asymptomatic, but local symptoms such as heartburn and dysphagia may be caused after local morphologic changes (e.g. strictures, ulcers, and fistulas). Moreover, malignant progression to esophageal adenocarcinoma or epithelial neoplasia may arise from HGM in exceedingly rare cases.

The size of esophageal HGM varies from 0.2 to 4 cm,[5] and the extent of HGM can vary from tiny microscopic foci to macroscopically apparent areas of red velvety patches (Fig. 7.1). The histology of HGM represents mostly a uniform fundictype, which contains parietal cells.[5,6] In less frequent cases, histological examination of HGM shows an "antral" pattern or a "transitional" cell type with fundic and antral glands. These types are mixed in some instances.[7] Chronic inflammation may be present and varies in extent (Fig. 7.2).

The malignant transformation of HGM is an exceedingly rare event compared to its high prevalence. Presumably, the heterotopic

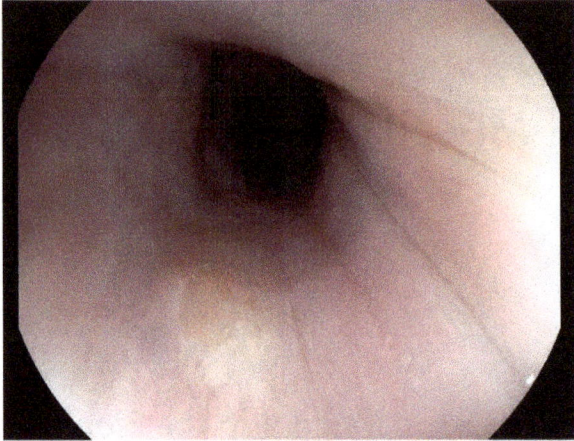

Fig. 7.1. White-light endoscopic view of a small reddish patch localized in the upper esophagus.

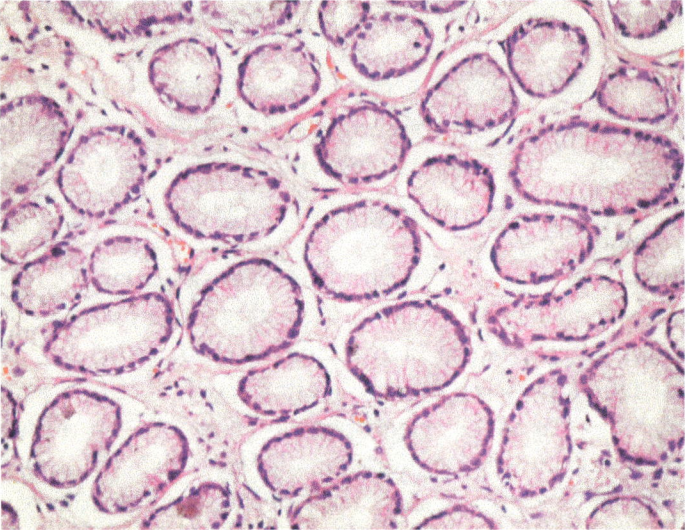

Fig. 7.2. The corresponding histopathology shows well-differentiated gastric tissue with mucus-secreting columnar cells, parietal cells, and chief cells.

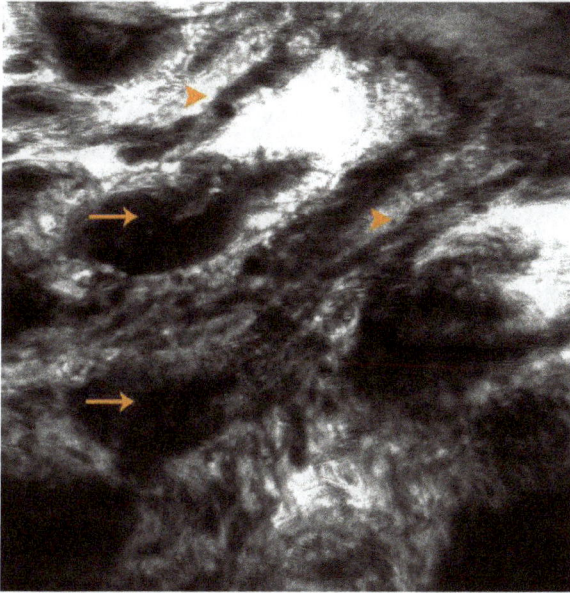

Fig. 7.3. Endomicroscopic imaging shows regularly arranged glands with round or oval openings (*arrows*); the columnar epithelial cells retain normal polarity; regularly shaped capillaries are identifiable in the stroma (*arrowheads*).

gastric epithelium may initially change to low and then high grade intraepithelial neoplasia, and finally progress to invasive carcinoma.

As with the histological findings, endomicroscopic imaging of HGM displays regularly arranged glands and evenly distributed columnar cells. Increased fluorescein leakage may be observed in inflammatory HGM (Figs. 7.3 and 7.4). Theoretically, the neoplastic changes could be differentiated from normal HGM, as has been described in Barrett's associated neoplasias.

Vascular Malformation of the Esophagus

Fluorescein sodium, as the routinely applied contrast agent for CLE examination, enables clear visualization of not only living cells and tissue, but also the vasculature of the mucosal layer in the GI tract during ongoing endoscopy. The high quality endomicroscopic imaging of the

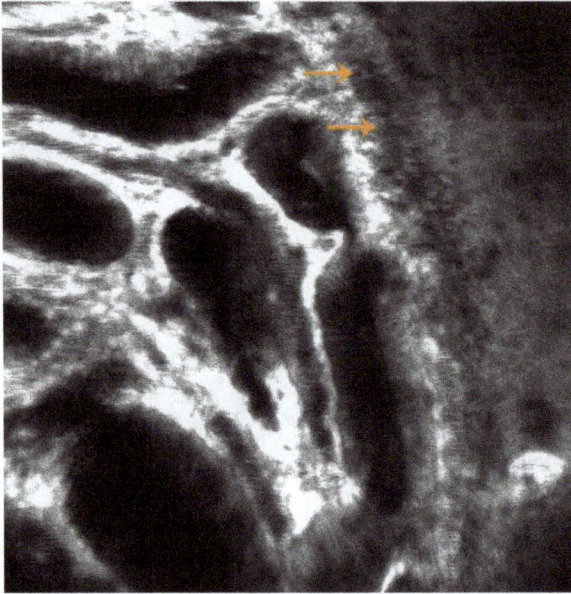

Fig. 7.4. The squamocolumnar junction is easily recognizable in the endomicroscopic image (*arrows*). The left side is the columnar epithelium with well-differentiated gastric glands, and the right side is the normal squamous epithelium.

vascular networks is almost a real-time angiography of the GI tract. Different characteristics of the microvascular architecture have been identified in normal and malignant lesions of the upper GI tract during confocal imaging.[8]

Here, we present a case report of a 59-year-old man who was examined by CLE. This patient was referred to the endoscopy unit for health examination and a local coarse mucosa was detected at the distal esophagus (Fig. 7.5). Endomicroscopic imaging of this area showed obviously distorted capillaries with an increased caliber (Figs. 7.6 and 7.7), and the final histological diagnosis was esophageal vascular malformation (Fig. 7.8).

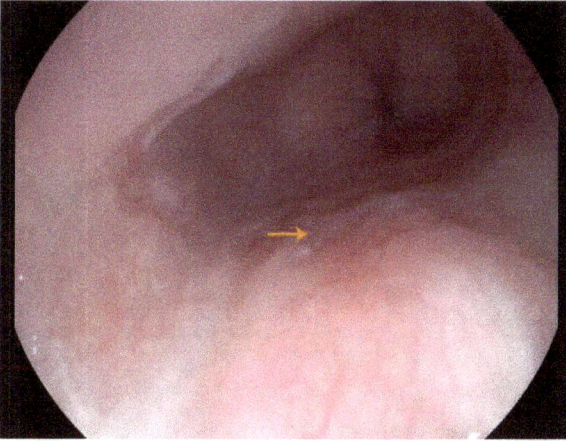

Fig. 7.5. A coarse patch is observed in the lower esophagus during white-light endoscopic imaging (*arrow*).

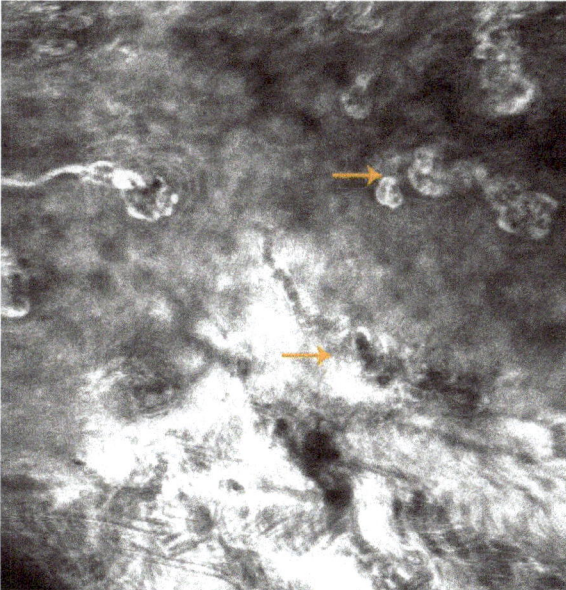

Fig. 7.6. In the upper part of this area, endomicroscopy shows prominent increased and distorted intracapillary papillary loops (*arrows*).

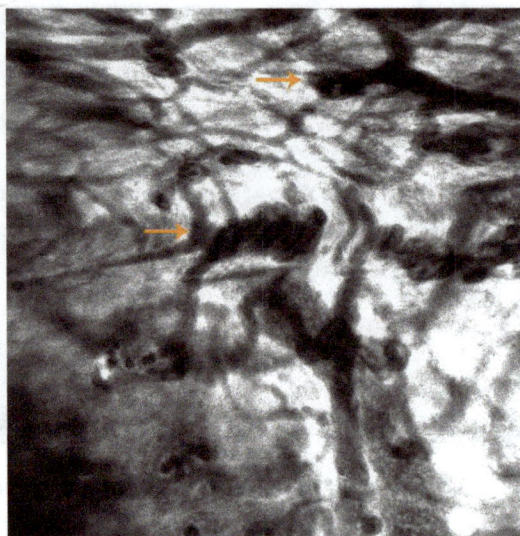

Fig. 7.7.   In the deeper part of this area, endomicroscopy shows even more vascular density and irregular appearance. These vessels display black configurations, which is different from the IPCLs, suggesting submucosal vessels (*arrows*).

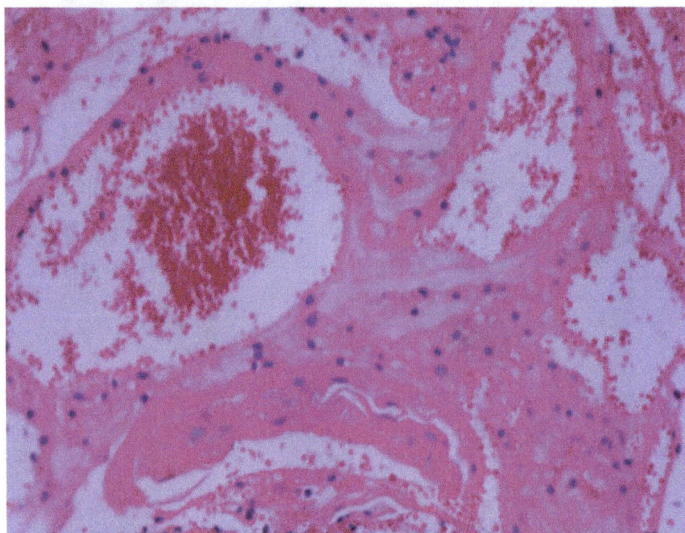

Fig. 7.8.   Histology shows malformation of the submucosal vessels, as with the endomicroscopic imaging.

References

1. De Angelis P, Trecca A, Francalanci P, *et al.* (2004) Heterotopic gastric mucosa of the rectum. *Endoscopy* **36**: 927.
2. Mann NS, Mann SK, Rachut E. (2000) Heterotopic gastric tissue in the duodenal bulb. *J Clin Gastroenterol* **30**: 303–306.
3. Caruso ML, Marzullo F. (1988) Jejunal adenocarcinoma in congenital heterotopic gastric mucosa. *J Clin Gastroenterol* **10**: 92–94.
4. Xeropotamos N, Skopelitou AS, Batsis C, Kappas AM. (2001) Heterotopic gastric mucosa together with intestinal metaplasia and moderate dysplasia in the gall bladder: report of two clinically unusual cases with literature review. *Gut* **48**: 719–723.
5. Ueno J, Davis SW, Tanakami A, *et al.* (1994) Ectopic gastric mucosa in the upper esophagus: detection and radiographic findings. *Radiology* **191**: 751–753.
6. Cox AJ, McClave SA. (1992) Incidence of heterotopic gastric mucosa in the upper esophagus. *Gastrointest Endosc* **38**: 108–109.
7. Jacobs E, Dehou MF. (1997) Heterotopic gastric mucosa in the upper esophagus: a prospective study of 33 cases and review of literature. *Endoscopy* **29**: 710–715.
8. Liu H, Li YQ, Yu T, *et al.* (2008) Confocal endomicroscopy for *in vivo* detection of microvascular architecture in normal and malignant lesions of upper gastrointestinal tract. *J Gastroenterol Hepatol* **23**: 56–61.

Part 4

STOMACH

Chapter 8

Normal Gastric Mucosa

Under the microscope, the wall of the stomach is composed of four layers: mucosa, submucosa, muscularis propria, and serosa. The layer of mucosa can be subdivided into epithelium, lamina propria, and muscularis mucosa (Fig. 8.1).

The entire epithelium of the gastric mucosa is lined with a single layer of tall columnar cells with their basal nuclei covering the surface papillae, and also forms numerous gastric pits that are openings for the gastric glands. The thickness of the epithelium is variable, about 0.3–1.5 mm in different parts. These columnar cells are connected to each other by junctional complexes and lateral cell membrane interdigitation. The cytoplasm is full of mucin granules. The main role of these cells is secreting gastric mucus into the luminal surface of the epithelium to form a barrier to protect the stomach, which also acts as a lubricant.

Beneath the epithelium, tubular gastric glands are found which empty into the pits and reach down to the muscularis propria, with 3–5 glands opening into each gastric pit. Three types of glands are usually found in gastric mucosa: cardiac, gastric, and pyloric glands. These glands vary in length and cellular composition, according to where they are situated. The gastric glands are mostly tubular, with seldom branching glands divided into a neck, a body, and a base, which are mainly distributed in the fundus and body zone. They have the greatest numbers in the stomach, and contain several types of cells: parietal cell, chief cell, neck mucous cell, stem cell, and endocrine cell. The cardiac glands are mainly distributed in the cardia, which is 1–4 cm downward from the gastroesophageal junction, and have no specific

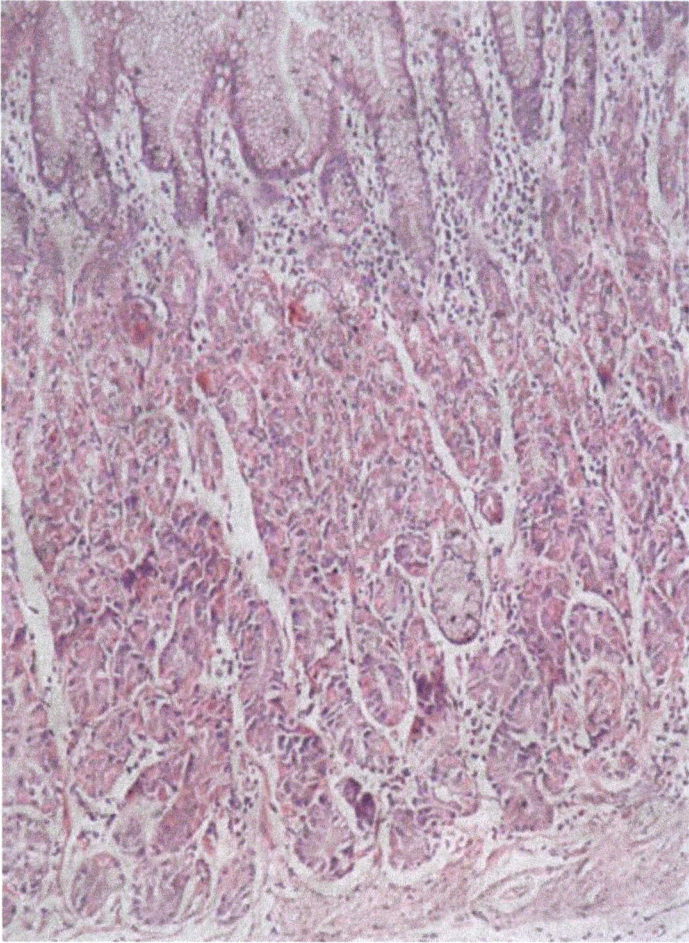

Fig. 8.1. Longitudinal section of gastric mucosa, HE × 100. The gastric mucosa comprises the epithelium, lamina propria, and muscularis mucosa. The epithelium is lined by surface mucous cells, which form the gastric pits. The lamina propria is filled by tubular glands with little connective tissue among them. The muscularis mucosa contains a layer of smooth muscle cells.

boundary with the gastric glands. They are composed mostly of mucous cells and little endocrine cells, and are mostly compound or branching tubular and tend to be grouped in lobules, with much smaller numbers but a bigger lumen compared with the gastric glands.

The pyloric glands occupy an area about 4–5 cm from the pylorus, which has much deeper gastric pits. They are also tubular glands but are not perpendicular to the surface, and are often branched and coiled in the deeper zone. Mainly mucous cells are found, with much more endocrine and stem cells and less parietal cells than the gastric glands. In particular, the pyloric glands contain a kind of goblet cells, which can secrete gastrin (Figs. 8.2 and 8.3.)

Except for tubular glands, the lamina propria contains numerous cells of the immune system, migrant cells from the blood, and resident loose connective tissue cells. Within the connective tissues, capillaries are distributed extensively and form a network supplying abundant blood for the stomach wall. Smooth muscle cells originating from the muscularis mucosa can also be seen in the lamina propria.

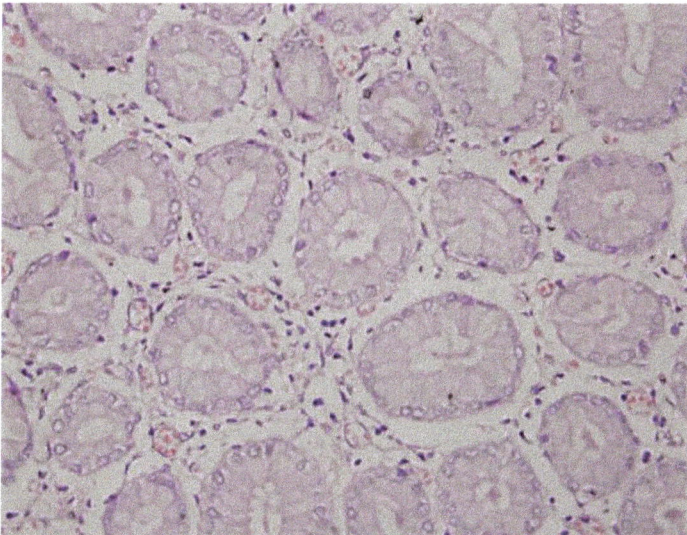

Fig. 8.2. Transverse section of a superficial gastric mucosa layer, HE × 400. (A) The round gastric pits are lined with a single layer of tall columnar cells with nuclei close to the basal membrane, and these pits are arranged regularly, with uniform size and shape. The interstitium between the gastric pits is mostly loose connective tissue; cells of the immune system and capillaries can also be seen.

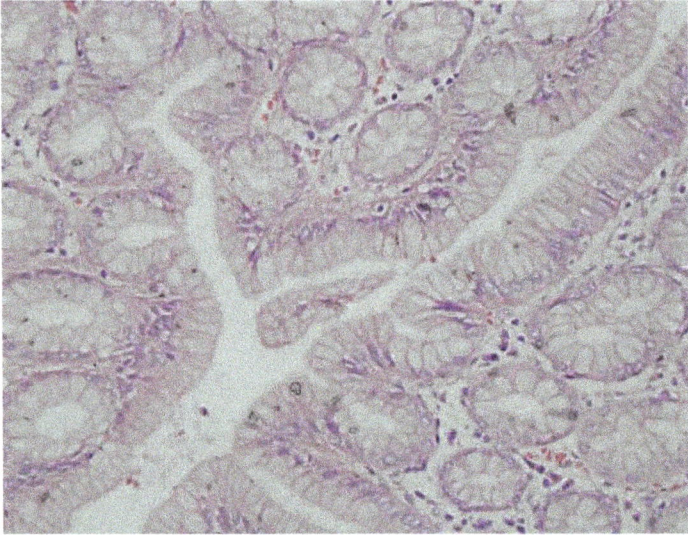

Fig. 8.2(B).   Several pits appear as irregular branching foveolars, while the rest are still round. Surface mucous cells can be seen in the surface of the gastric pits.

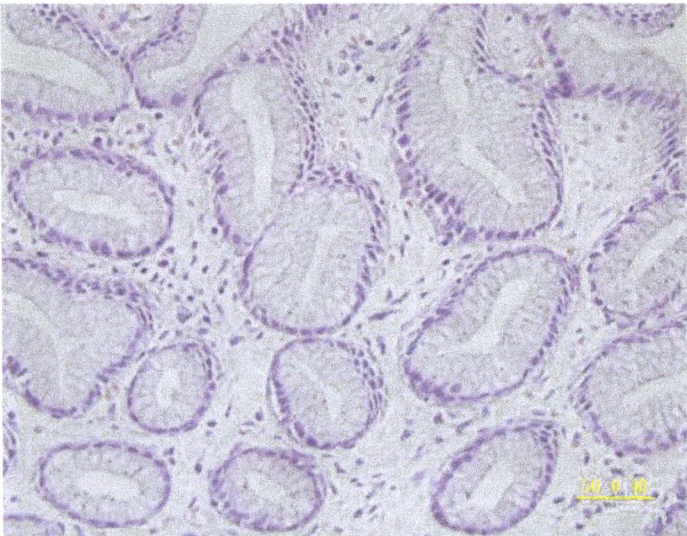

Fig. 8.2(C).   Due to the different section of cutting, the epithelial cells appear stratified but with normal structure, which needs to be distinguished from atypical hyperplasia of epithelium.

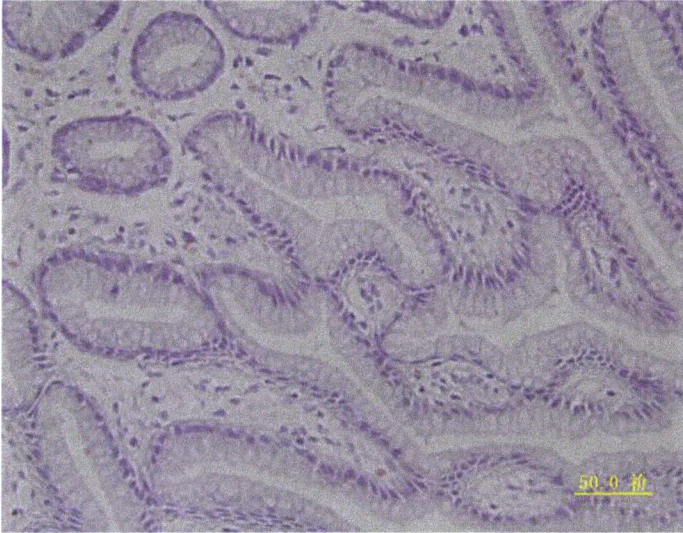

Fig. 8.2(D).   Gastric pits with long continuous rod-like and branched shape.

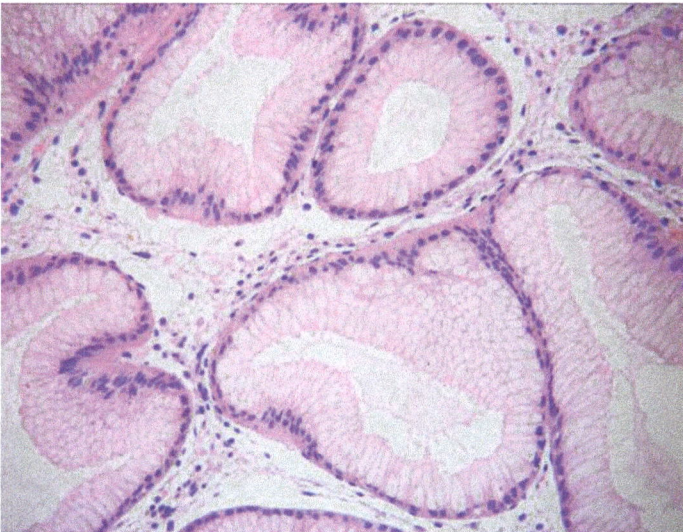

Fig. 8.3.   Transverse section of a deep gastric mucosa layer, HE × 400. (A) Cardiac glands are mostly tubular mucous glands with much bigger lumens and smaller numbers. The nuclei of the mucous cells are sitting in the basal part, and the cytoplasm is full of mucous granules which stain a little in HE staining.

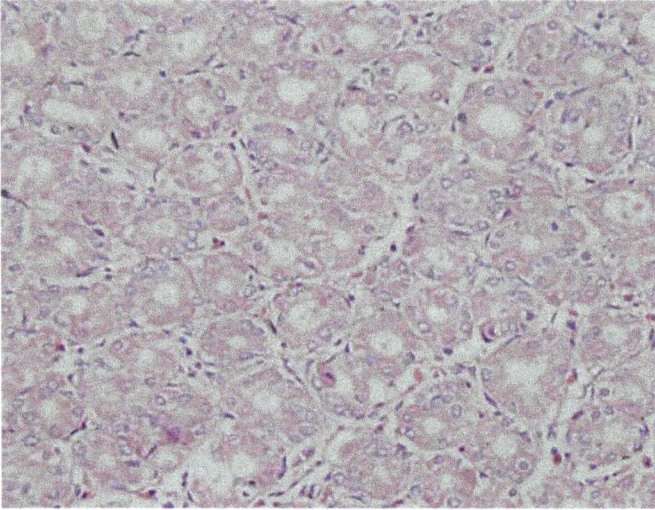

Fig. 8.3(B).   Gastric glands in the body of the stomach have a tight arrangement, seldom with connective tissues between the glands. Mainly parietal cells and chief cells are included.

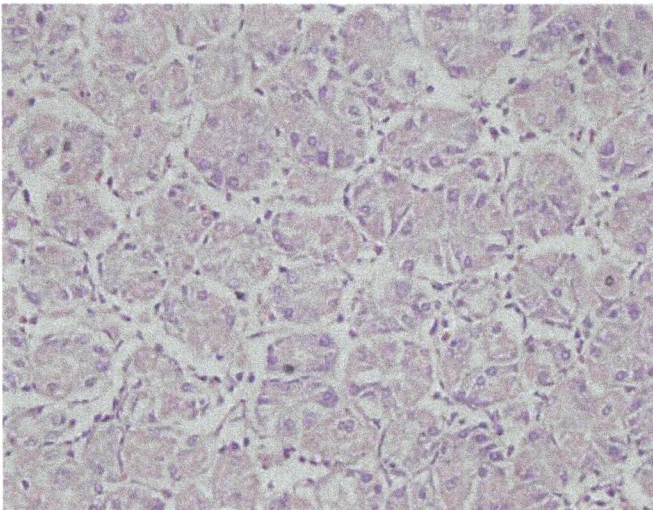

Fig. 8.3(C).   The chief cells become primary in the gastric glands in the fundus part, while few parietal cells are found here. The round nuclei are in the basal part, and the basal cytoplasm is basophilic, and is stained red in HE staining.

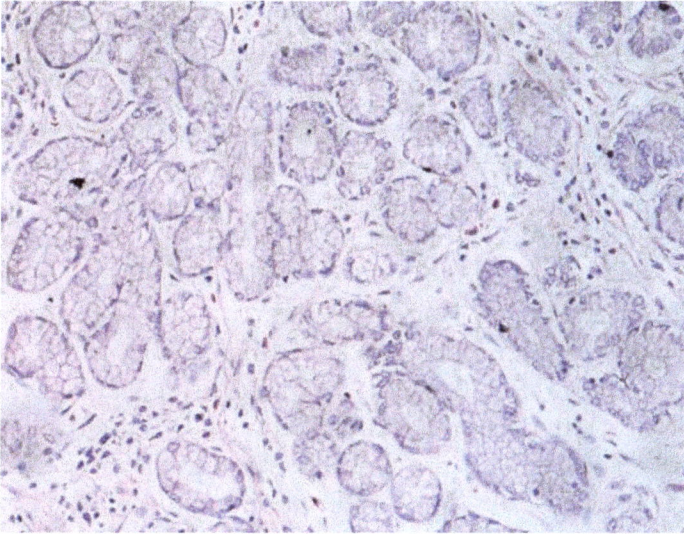

Fig. 8.3(D). Pyloric glands are usually branched tubular mucous glands, and are lightly stained in HE staining.

Endomicroscopic Imaging of Normal Gastric Mucosa

Confocal endomicroscopy produces high magnification images of surface and subsurface tissues of the GI tract at the cellular level, and the epithelium, the structure of gastric pits, and the interstitium between the pits can be clearly visualized. After IV administration of the fluorescein sodium, the columnar epithelium looks like a tiled mosaic of cells in the normal stomach. In normal mucosa, the epithelium is intact without effusion of fluorescein, and the epithelial cells are arranged regularly like paving stones. Among the columnar cells, the dark parts are the openings of gastric pits. As mentioned before, the shape of gastric pits varies with different gland types.

The gastric pits are the basic units of the microstructures on the surface of gastric mucosa. In the stomach, the architecture of the gastric pits was observed as small invaginations. By inspecting the pit pattern, we can distinguish the different types of glands, or normal mucosa from inflammatory or neoplastic mucosa. In the normal mucosa with fundic glands, round gastric pits with approximately uniform shape and size can be found with a cobblestone appearance in superficial CLE images, and the epithelial cells are regularly arranged between the pits. The subsurface (below superficial epithelial cells) gastric pits showed a honeycomb-like appearance. The interstitium between gastric pits can be seen clearly; the bright parts are capillaries. In the surface of normal mucosa with pyloric glands, the foveolars appear continuous short rod-like, with approximately uniform length. The subsurface gastric pits are long and more slit-like, and the coil-shaped blood vessels can be seen in the interstitium, and sometimes the erythrocytes (black dots) can be visualized in the lumen of the vessels. The width of the interstitium between the subsurface pits and that of the pits themselves are about the same. In the caporal the foveolars are noncontinuous short rod-like, while in the antral mucosa the pits appear elongated and tortuous branchlike (Figs. 8.4–8.6)

The mucous layer cannot be completely scanned by confocal endosmicroscopy, because the depth of scanning is only 250 μm while the thickness of the mucosa is 300–1500 μm. The current study demonstrated that confocal endomicroscopy was able to visualize

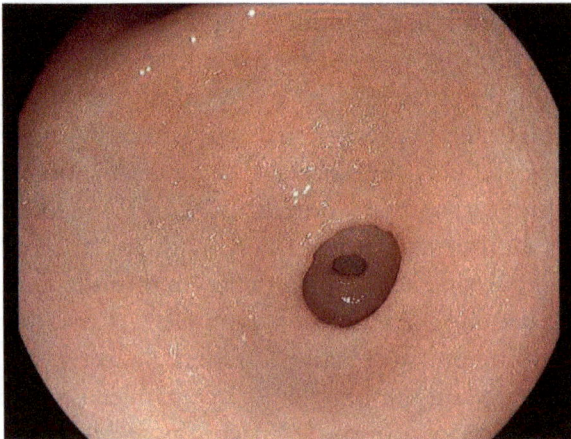

Fig. 8.4.(A)   Normal mucosa in the corpus of the stomach. (A) Under conventional white-light endoscopy, normal gastric mucosa is light orange in color, and appears thin and lubricious.

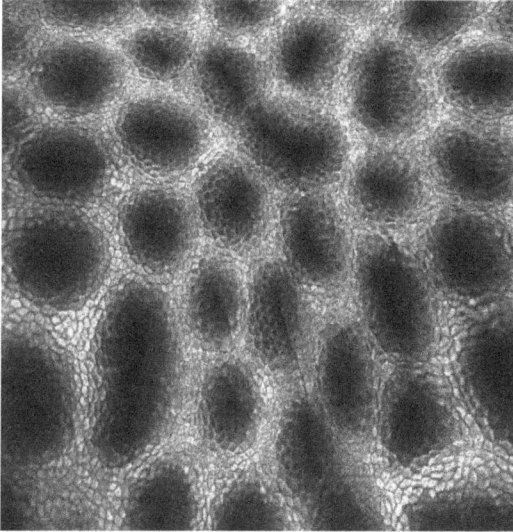

Fig. 8.4(B). Superficial CLE image of normal mucosa with fundic glands: round gastric pits with approximately uniform shape and size can be found with a cobble-stone appearance. The gastric pits are lined with a layer of paving-stone-like columnar cells, and their openings are the dark parts of the image.

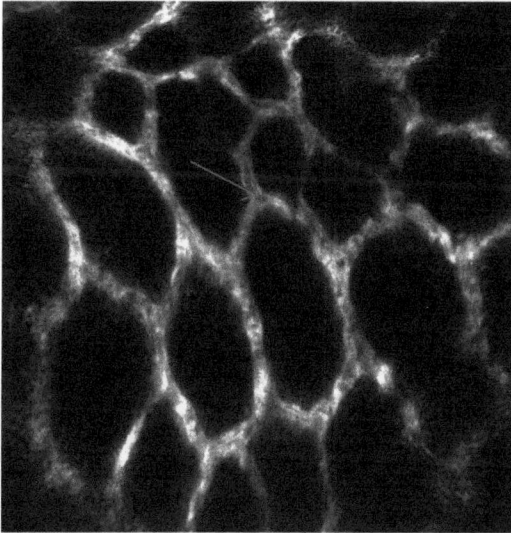

Fig. 8.4(C). Deep CLE image of normal mucosa with fundic glands: the subsurface gastric pits show a honeycomb-like appearance. The interstitium between gastric pits can be seen clearly; the bright parts are capillaries (*red arrow*).

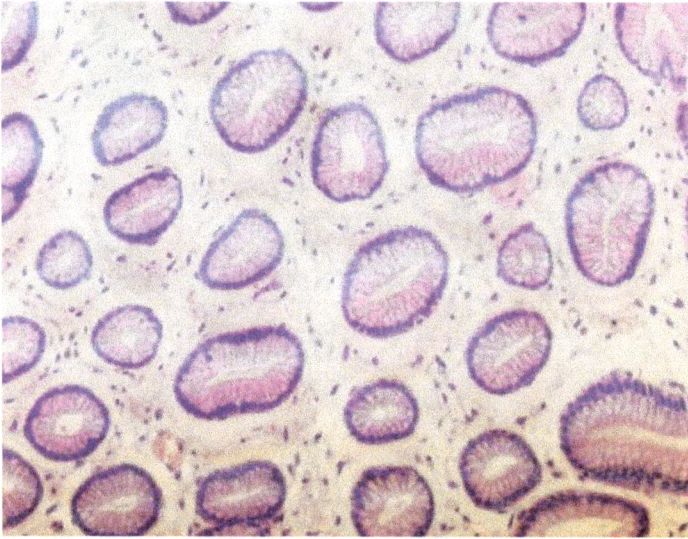

Fig. 8.4(D).   Corresponding histological image of the transverse section (HE × 400).

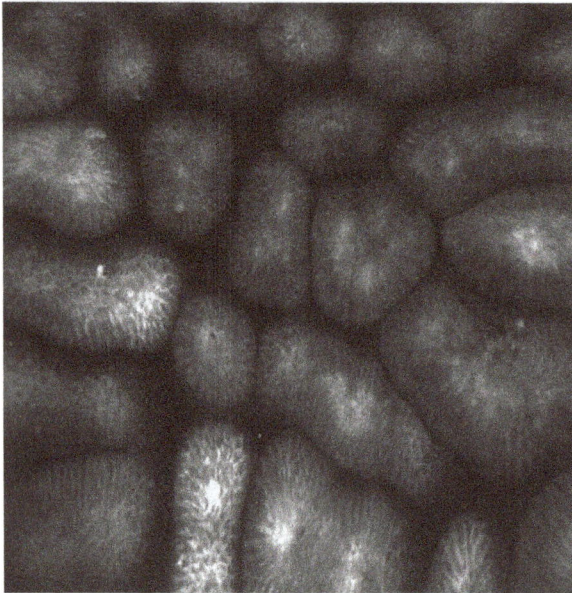

Fig. 8.5.   Normal mucosa in the fundus of the stomach. (A) Superficial CLE image of normal mucosa with pyloric glands: the foveolars appear continuous short rod-like, with approximately uniform length and with slitlike openings.

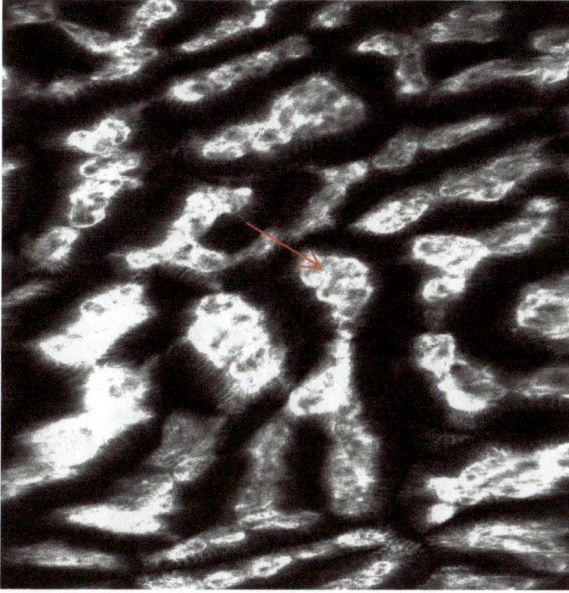

Fig. 8.5(B). Deep CLE image of normal mucosa with pyloric glands: the subsurface gastric pits are long and more slit-like, and coil-shaped blood vessels can be seen in the interstitium (*red arrow*).

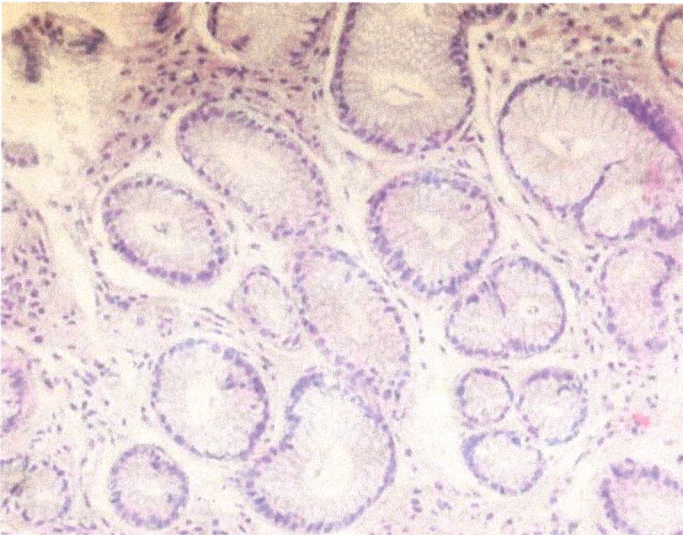

Fig. 8.5(C). Corresponding histological image of the transverse section (HE × 400).

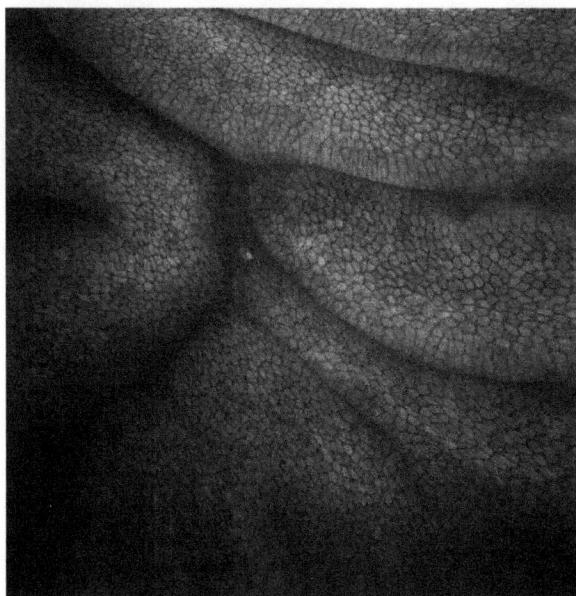

Fig. 8.6.   CLE image of mucosa with pyloric glands after spraying of acriflavine. The continuous short rod-like foveolars are clearly visualized.

precisely the epithelium, the structure of the pit, and the pit pattern of normal mucosa. However, the structures beneath the lamina propria layer, like submucosa and muscularis propria, limit inspection.

References

1. Kiesslich R, Galle PR, Neurath MF. (2008) *Atlas of Endomicroscopy.* Springer Medizin Verlag.
2. Day DW, Jass JR, Price AB, *et al.* (2002) *Morson and Dawson's Gastrointestinal Pathology,* 4th ed.
3. Zhang J-N, Li Y-Q, Zhao Y-A. (2008) Classification of gastric pit patterns by confocal endomicroscopy. *Gastrointest Endosc* **67**: 843–853.

Chapter 9

Gastritis

Chronic gastritis is defined as the inflammatory reaction of gastric mucosa, which is caused by various injury factors. The updated Sydney system provides three major categories: nonatrophic gastritis, atrophic gastritis, and special forms of gastritis. Histologically, five morphological variables (*H. pylori* density, activity, chronic inflammation, glandular atrophy, and intestinal metaplasia) must be classified, because of the relationship to their associated diseases.[1] To some extent, with 500–1000-time magnification by CLE, *in vivo* visualization of the five variables can be achieved.

Nonatrophic Gastritis

Nonatrophic gastritis has many endoscopic features, such as edema, erythema (punctate or confluent), erosion, and exudates. However, several studies have indicated that these endoscopic features are not always in line with corresponding histological findings.[2] Therefore, accurate diagnosis of chronic gastritis should be confirmed by histological examination. Because epithelial cells and subepithelial structures can be clearly identified, nonatrophic gastritis has specific features under CLE, in which the graded variables of *H. pylori* infection, activity, and chronic inflammation are introduced.

H. pylori Infection

Observation of the H. pylori organism

The organism of *H. pylori* usually colonizes on the surface and gastric upper pits of the epithelium, which makes observing *H. pylori* possible under CLE. In addition to nucleus dyeing, acriflavine can also label the organism because of its take-up by *H. pylori*.[3] In CLE images, large groups of *H. pylori* organisms appear as clusters of white spots within the lumen of pits, and even individual bacteria (separate white spots) could be recognized (Fig. 9.1).[4] More often, we are not able to detect *H. pylori* bacteria in the gastric mucosa showing intestinal metaplasia under CLE, which enables us to perform a targeted biopsy to detect *H. pylori* avoiding intestinal metaplasia.

H. *pylori–induced gastritis*

H. pylori plays a major role in more than one type of nonautoimmune chronic gastritis. It can cause damage to gastric epithelium such as mucosal edema and even cell shedding, neutrophil activity, and chronic inflammation, which can be clearly visualized by CLE.

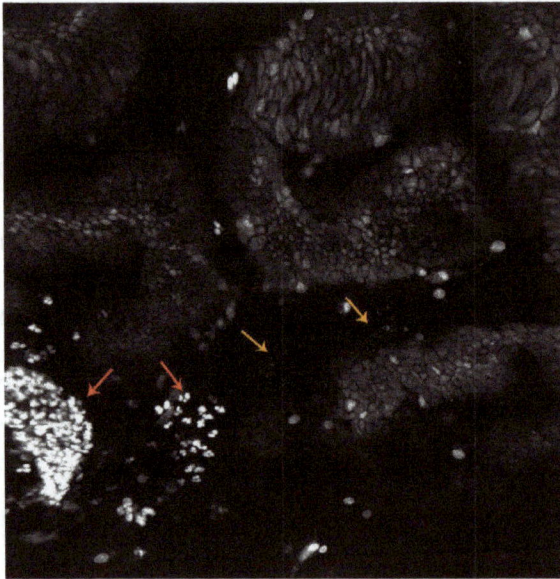

Fig. 9.1(A). Appearance of *H. pylori* organisms in a CLE image. Clusters of white spots can be seen in the lumen of gastric pits (*orange arrows*), accompanied by neutrophil infiltration (*red arrows*).

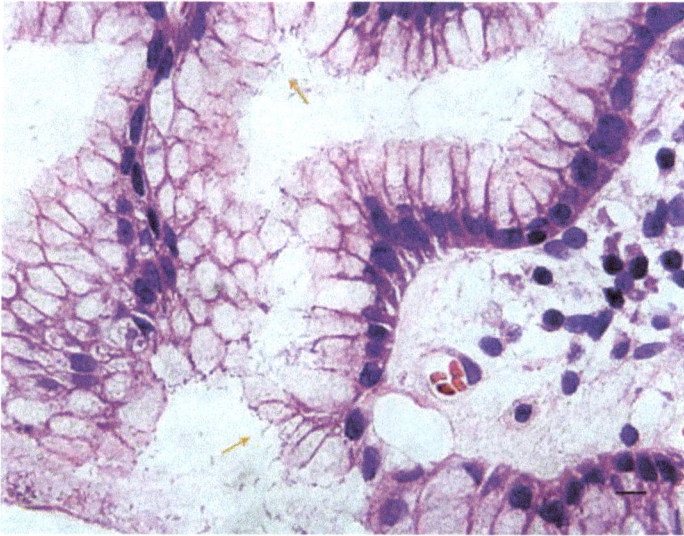

Fig. 9.1(B). Corresponding histological images for *H. pylori* infection (×400, H&E). The short rodlike organisms colonized along the pit edge can be clearly identified using routine hematoxylin and eosin staining (*orange arrow*).

Mucosal edema

Mucosal edema manifests in the gastric epithelium as widening of the intercellular spaces, change of cell color (gray to dark), and change of cell shape (polygonal to round). Possibly because of the increased permeability, when one is using fluorescein staining (concentration of 10%), fluorescein leakage into the intercellular spaces which shows a white ring surrounding the cells can be clearly seen by CLE (Fig. 9.2).

Cell shedding

Cell shedding is a consequent event after gastric epithelial cell degeneration or excessive apoptosis, which are mostly induced by some *H. pylori*–secreted toxins, such as Vac A toxin, Cag A toxin, and urease. With fluorescein staining, the gaps caused by cell shedding are usually filled with white fluorescein (Fig. 9.3).

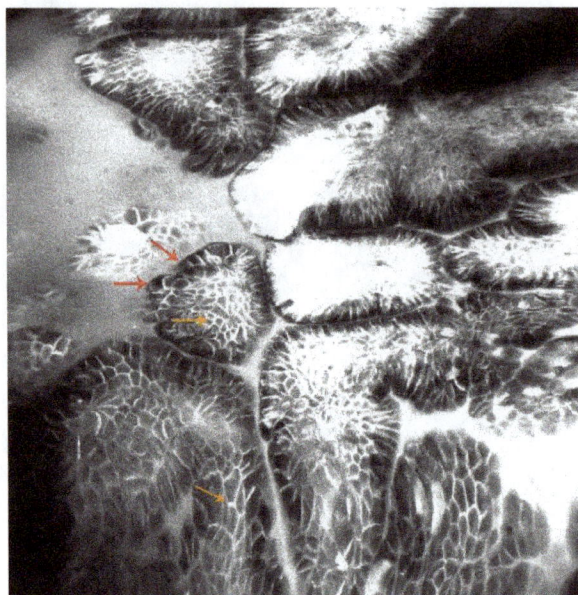

Fig. 9.2. Endomicroscopic appearance of mucosal edema in the antrum (10% fluorescein staining). The intercellular spaces are wider and brighter than the normal state, which shows a white ring surrounding the cells (orange arrows). The epithelial cells are slightly swollen and become darker than normal (red arrows).

Neutrophil activity

The presence of neutrophils is a diagnostic marker of acute inflammation or so-called activity in *H. pylori*–induced chronic gastritis. Neutrophils (particularly within the foveolar lumen) can be easily seen in CLE images by means of acriflavine dyeing, because the nucleus can be dyed by acriflavine other than fluorescein. *H. pylori* organisms are frequently found in the CLE images in which neutrophils are present. As with the Sydney system, the severity of neutrophil activity can be classified by CLE. With marked activity, pit abscesses can be seen (Fig. 9.4).

Chronic inflammation (lymphocyte infiltration)

Chronic inflammation is a basic feature of various forms of chronic gastritis, especially lymphocytic gastritis and *H. pylori*-induced gastritis.

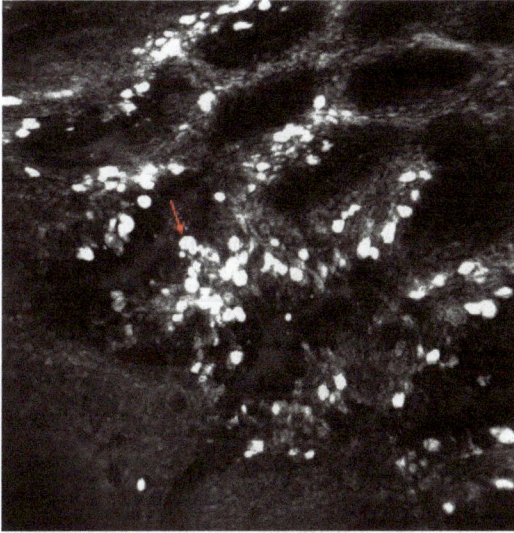

Fig. 9.3. *H. pylori-associated* cell shedding by CLE (10% fluorescein staining). The gaps left after cell degeneration or apoptosis are usually filled with fluorescein, showing white and round spots (*red arrow*).

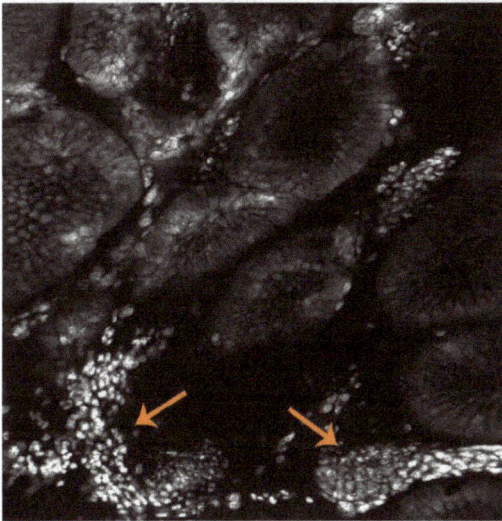

Fig. 9.4. Pit abscesses in a CLE image (0.02% acriflavine staining). A mass of neutrophils in the pit lumen form pit abscesses, indicating marked activity (*orange arrows*).

Table 9.1.   Classification of the Gastric Pit Pattern in Chronic Inflammation

	Antrum	Corpus
Chronic inflammation	Elongated and tortuous branch-like pits	Noncontinuous short rod-like pits
Moderate to marked activity	Widened interstitium between two pits	Dilated lumens of gastric pits
	Defect of topical epithelial cells of pits	Defect of topical epithelial cells of pits

However, lymphocyte infiltration is difficult to visualize directly by CLE, because of some limitations. The major reason is that the confocal laser scanning cannot reach enough depth of the gastric mucosa, and the lymphocytic nucleus is hard to reveal by either fluorescein or acriflavine dyeing. But there are many indirect signs shown by CLE that can predict the severity of gastric chronic inflammation accurately. There are various forms of gastric pits — gastric pit patterns that may be changed by chronic inflammatory cell infiltration. According to Zhang *et al.*'s reports,[5] the gastric pit pattern specific for inflammatory alteration can be classified respectively into the gastric antrum and corpus (Table 9.1). In the gastric antrum, the normal continuous short rod-like pits will change to elongated and tortuous branch-like pits when chronic inflammation exists. Similarly, in the gastric corpus, the normal round pits will change to noncontinuous short rod-like pits when chronic inflammation exists. Furthermore, in a background of chronic inflammation, the presence of *H. pylori* and neutrophils will damage the epithelium and glands, manifested as mucosal edema, cell shedding, and even intraepithelial neutrophils and/or lymphocytes (Fig. 9.5).

Atrophic Gastritis

Atrophic gastritis includes glandular atrophy and metaplasia histologically. Glandular atrophy is manifested as loss of glandular tissue, which may result from erosion or ulceration or a prolonged inflammatory process. Metaplasia mostly refers to the gastric mucosa being replaced by intestinal tissues, which carries an increased risk of gastric cancer.

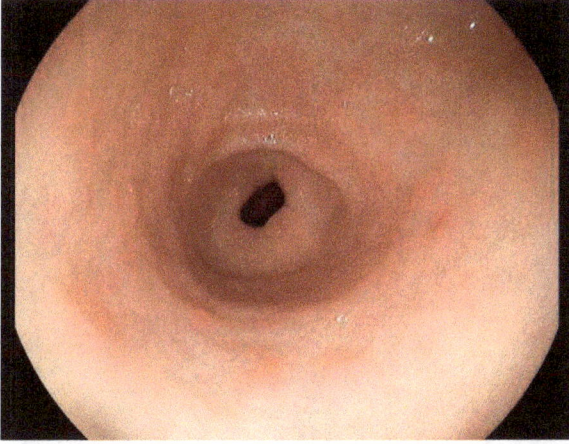

Fig. 9.5(A).   High-resolution white-light endoscopy indicating mild chronic antral gastritis. Mucosal edema and sporadic erythema can be seen in the antrum.

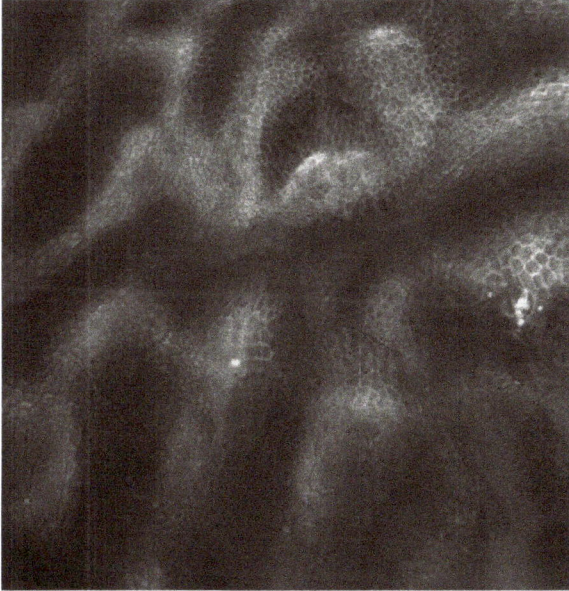

Fig. 9.5(B).   CLE features of mild chronic antral gastritis (10% fluoresein staining). Slightly elongated and tortuous branch-like pits are present and small numbers of epithelial cells become dark and even disappear. Focal fluorescein leakage can be seen in less than half of the visual field.

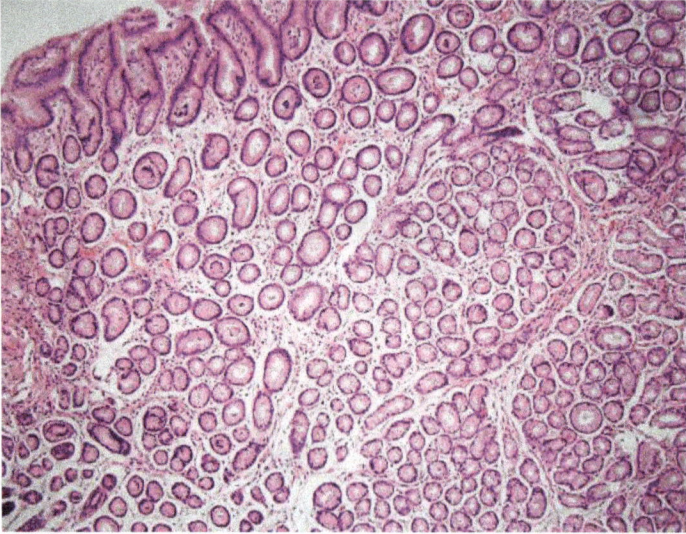

Fig. 9.5(C).   Histological image of mild inflammation (×200, H&E). Similar branch-like pits can be observed, with slightly increased inflammatory cells.

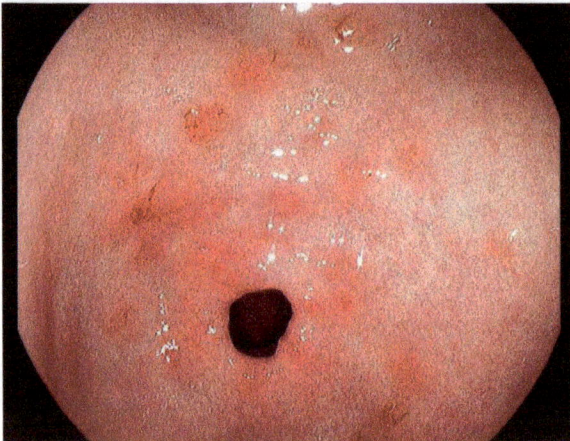

Fig. 9.5(D).   High-resolution white-light endoscopy indicating moderate to marked active inflammation in the antrum. Obvious edema, multiple erythemas, and erosive lesions appear surrounding the pylorus.

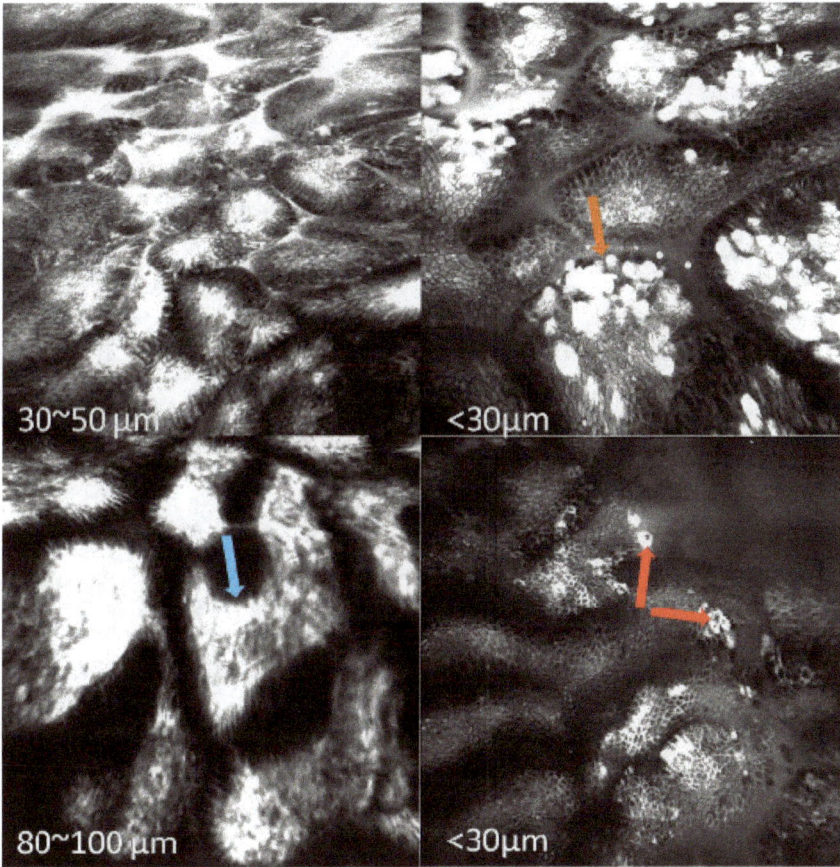

Fig. 9.5(E). CLE images of moderate to marked active inflammation at different depths and visual fields of the antrum (10% fluorescein staining). Markedly elongated and tortuous branchlike pits are present and large numbers of epithelial cells are damaged as shedding (*orange arrow*) or intraepithelial inflammatory cells (*red arrows*). Widespread fluorescein leakage can be seen in more than half of the visual field. Widened interstitium is appearing in the deeper layer of the mucosa (*blue arrow*).

The endoscopic atrophic gastritis is diagnosed when some pearly whitish mucosal discoloration appears, mucosa is thinning, and the vascular pattern becomes visible in the non-overdistended stomach.[6]

In autommune gastritis, diffuse glandular atrophy can usually be found in the absence of intestinal metaplasia in the corpus, so

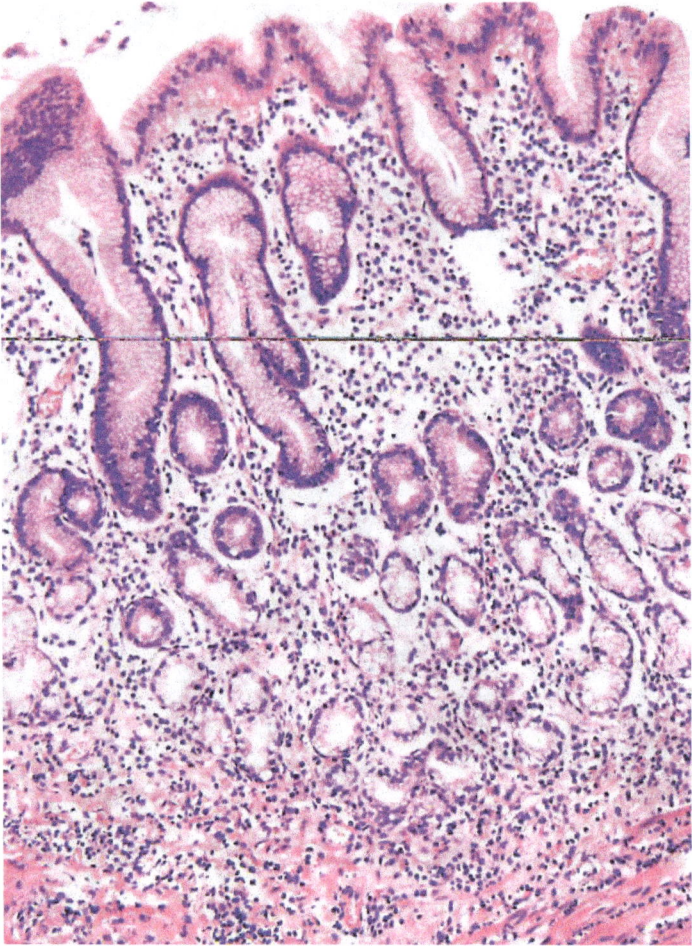

Fig. 9.5(F).   Histological image of marked active inflammation in the antrum (×200, H&E). Significantly increased inflammatory cells can be seen present in the full layer of the mucosa accompanied by degenerated epithelium and destroyed dilated pits.

glandular atrophy and metaplasia should be evaluated and graded independently.

Direct visualization of the loss of glandular tissue by CLE is also difficult, because the confocal laser can only penetrate a thickness of 250 μm of the mucosa and the cross-sectional CLE image provides

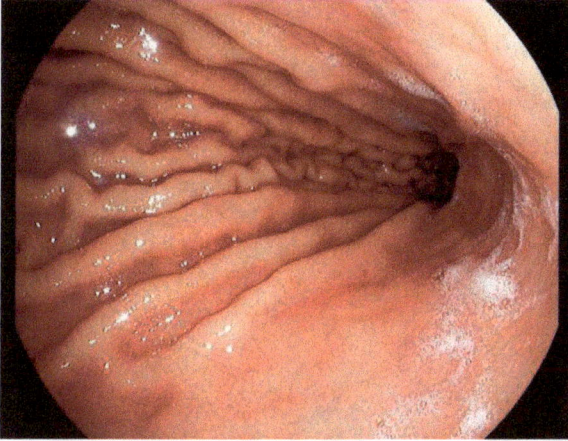

Fig. 9.5(G). High-resolution white-light endoscopy indicating mild gastric corporal inflammation. Mild congestion and edema can be seen in the corpus.

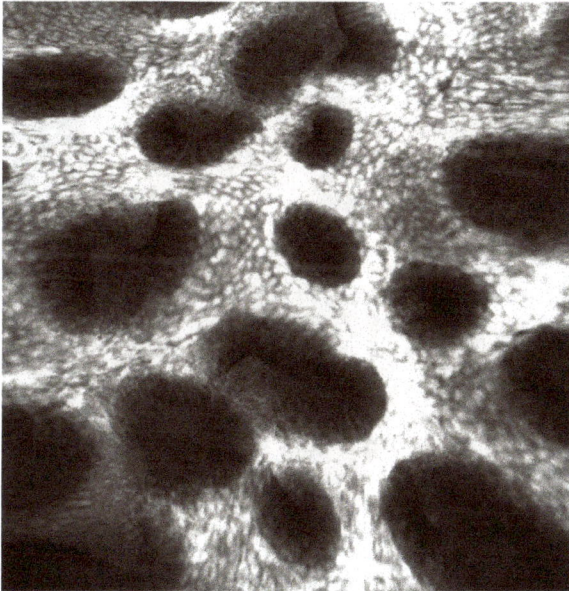

Fig. 9.5(H). CLE image of mild chronic corporal gastritis (10% fluorescein staining). Noncontinuous short rod-like pits and dark epithelial cells can be identified. Focal fluorescein leakage can be clearly observed.

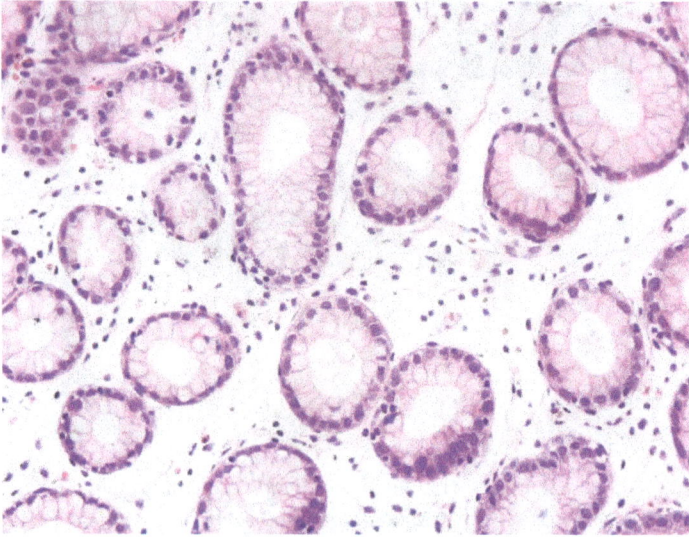

Fig. 9.5(I). Histological image of mild inflammation in the corpus (×400, H&E, cross section). Slightly distorted gastric pits and small numbers of inflammatory cells infiltration are within the shallow layer of the mucosa.

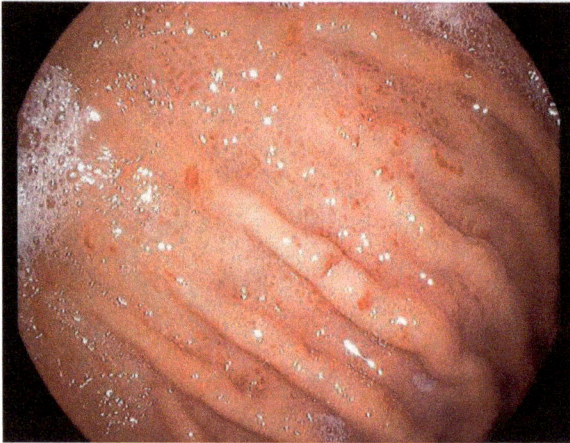

Fig. 9.5(J). High-resolution white-light endoscopy indicating moderate to marked gastric corporal active inflammation. A large quantity of erosive lesions and marked mucosal edema can be clearly visualized.

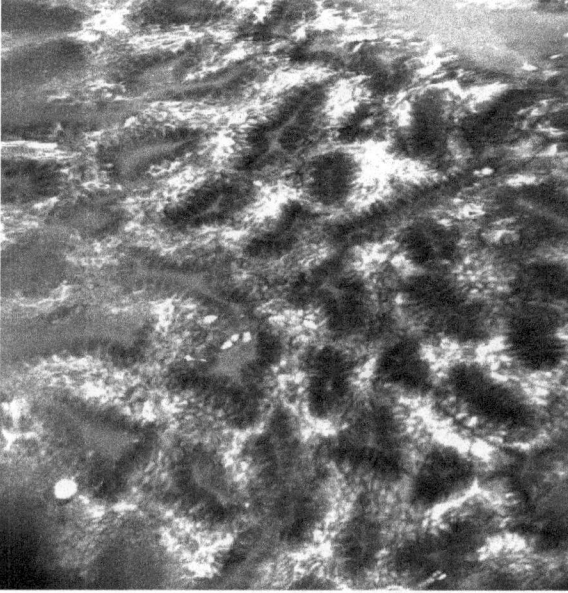

Fig. 9.5(K). CLE image of moderate to marked chronic corporal gastritis (10% fluorescein staining). Noncontinuous short rod-like pits are present with dilating openings. Epithelial cell damage is more frequent and fluorescein leakage is widespread.

limited information on distribution of the glandular tissue. However, the alteration of gastric pits, which is clearly shown by CLE, can predict the loss of glands accurately when atrophy occurs. In the aspect of intestinal metaplasia, goblet cells, the villiform shape of foveolar epithelium, columnar absorptive cells, and the brush border can directly be identified by CLE, which has a high accuracy in diagnosing intestinal metaplasia.[7]

Glandular atrophy

Endomicroscopically, glandular atrophy shows the alteration of gastric pits and microvascular architecture. Slight atrophy shows widened, sparse, and irregularly arranged gastric pits. Severe atrophy shows significantly reduced pits with enlarged openings and reduced subepithelial capillary networks with the shape changed (Fig. 9.6).

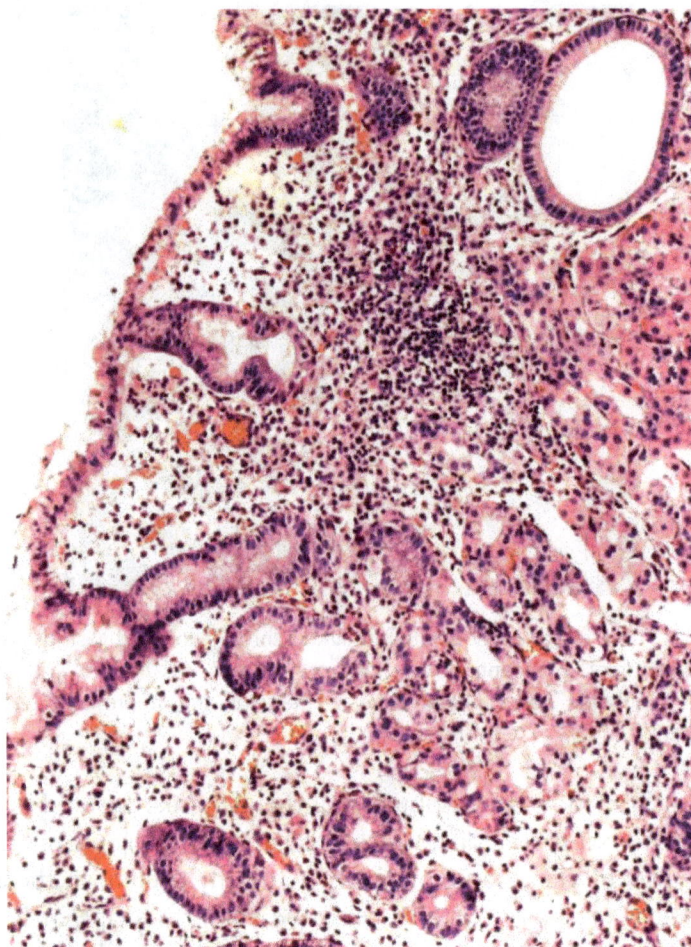

Fig. 9.5(L). Histological image of moderate to marked active inflammation in the corpus (×200, H&E). Significantly increased inflammatory cells infiltration into the full thickness of the mucosa can be seen. The gastric pits are distorted with dilated openings in a widened interstitium background.

Intestinal metaplasia

Gastric intestinal metaplasia is defined as the gastric epithelium being replaced by intestinal epithelium, which is generally regarded as a high cancer risk condition.[8] Histologically, the metaplastic

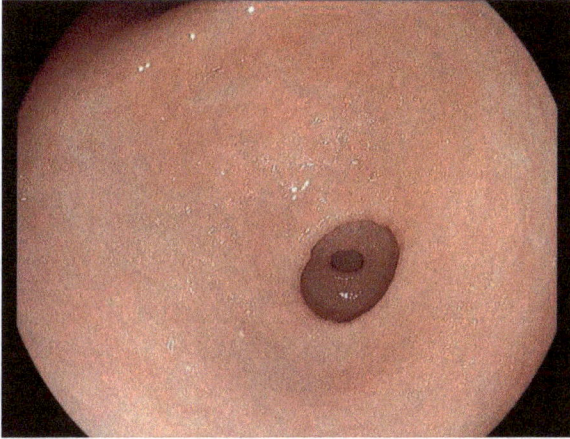

Fig. 9.6(A). High-resolution white-light endoscopy showing mild antral atrophy. Some pearly whitish mucosal discoloration is present and the vascular pattern becomes visible.

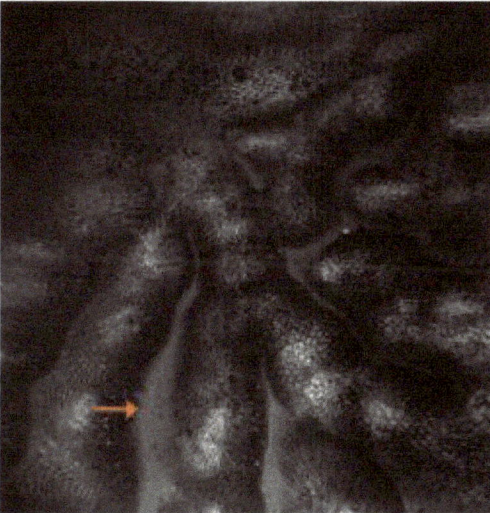

Fig. 9.6(B). CLE image of mild antral atrophy (10% fluorescein staining). The epithelial cells are regular, but the number of gastric pits decreases, with the openings slightly dilated (*orange arrow*).

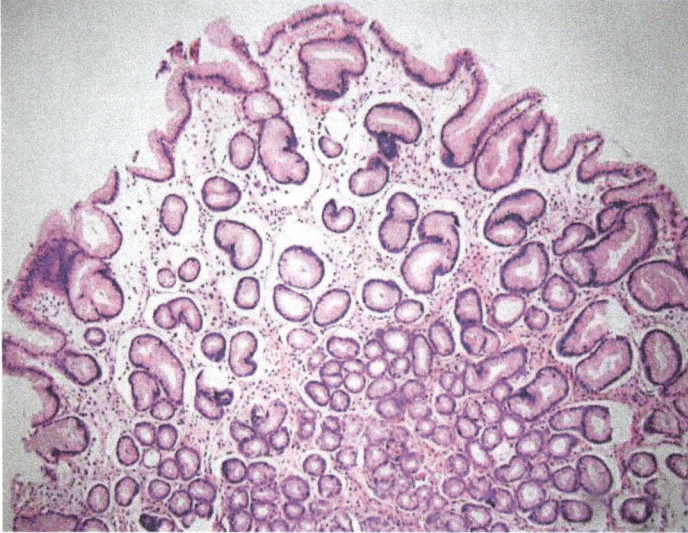

Fig. 9.6(C). Histological image of mild antral atrophy (×200, H&E). Decrease in the number of gastric pits and sparse distribution of gastric glands can be seen.

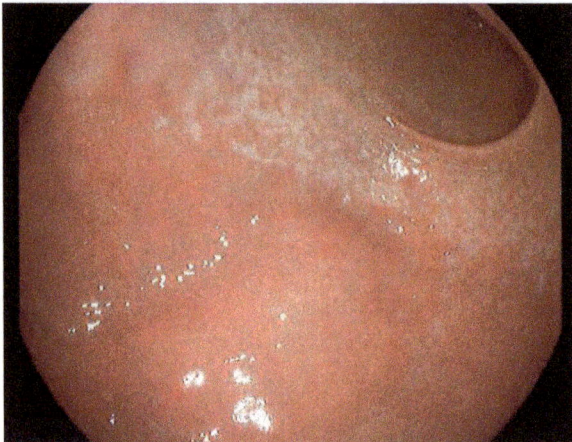

Fig. 9.6(D). High-resolution white-light endoscopy showing moderate to marked antral atrophy. The mucosa is rough and thinning, appearing as a granular pattern. A demarcation line between atrophic and nonatrophic mucosa can be clearly seen.

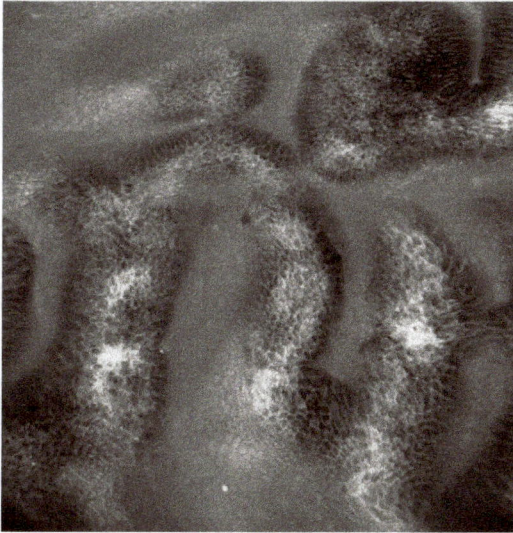

Fig. 9.6(E). Endomicroscopy of moderate to marked glandular atrophy in the gastric antrum (10% fluorescein staining). Significantly decreased gastric pits with dilated lumen (full of mucus) can be clearly visualized.

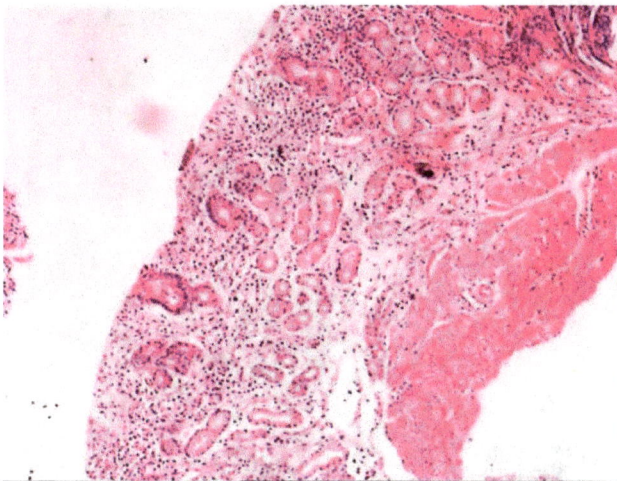

Fig. 9.6(F). Histological image of moderate to marked antral atrophy (×200, H&E). The specialized glands were significantly decreased and the gastric pits almost disappeared.

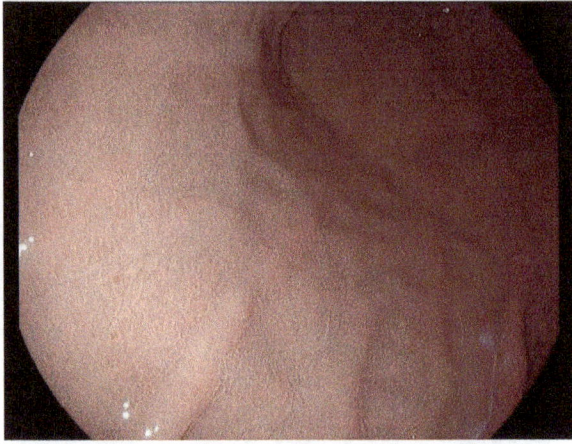

Fig. 9.6(G).   High-resolution white-light endoscopy showing mild corporal atrophy. Only the rough mucosa can be seen.

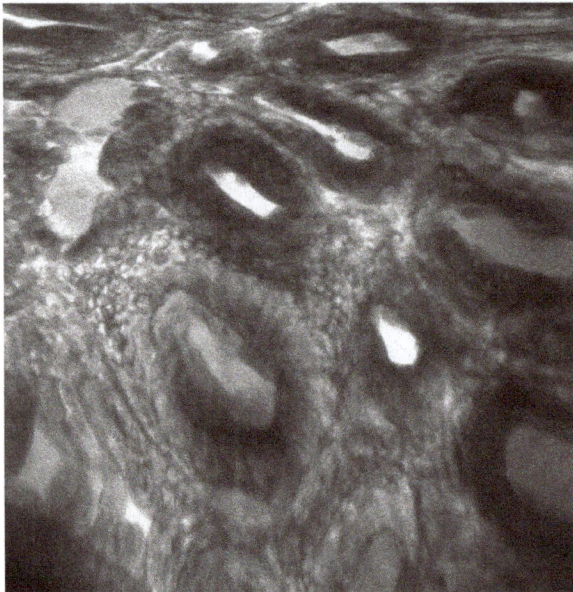

Fig. 9.6(H).   Corresponding endomicroscopy of mild glandular atrophy in the gastric corpus (10% fluorescein staining). The decreased gastric pits with dilated openings can be seen and fluorescein leakage is present.

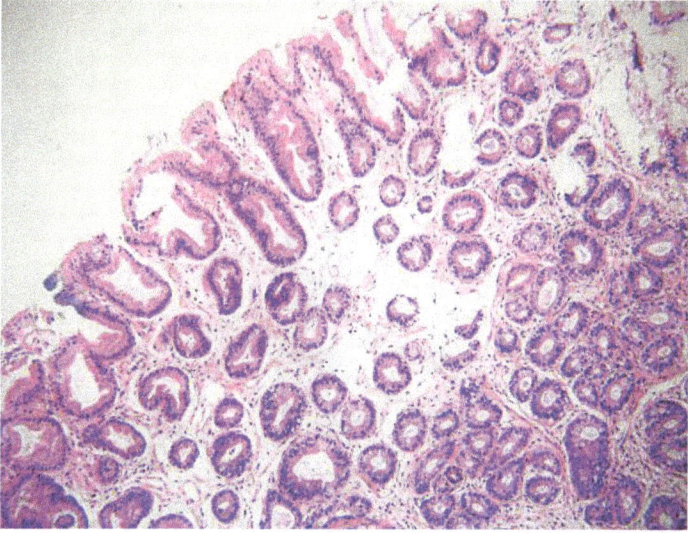

Fig. 9.6(I). Histological image of mild glandular atrophy in the gastric corpus (×200, H&E). Slightly decreased specialized glands can be seen.

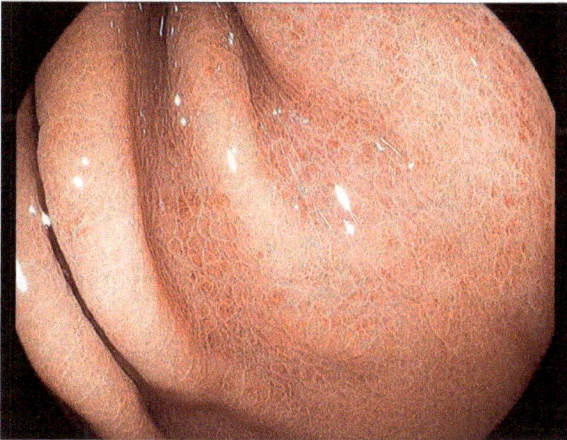

Fig. 9.6(J). High-resolution white-light endoscopy showing moderate to marked corporal atrophy. Obvious edema, erythema, and exudation can be found in the rough mucosa.

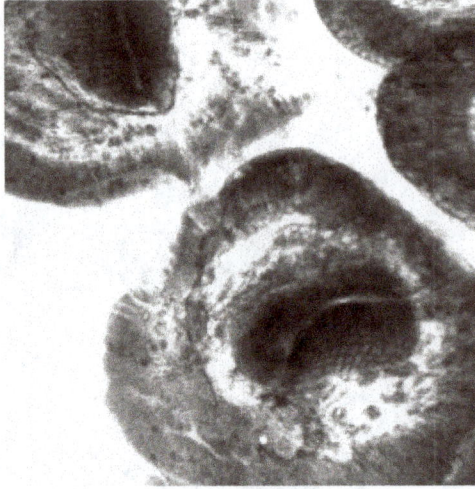

Fig. 9.6(K).   Enomicroscopy of moderate to marked glandular atrophy in the gastric corpus (10% fluorescein staining). The corporal pits are destroyed and significantly decreased, with the pit openings markedly dilated. Furthermore, subepithelial capillary networks disappear.

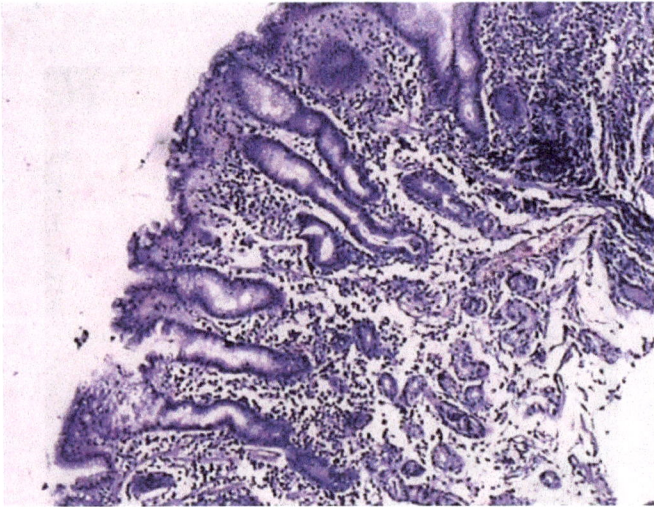

Fig. 9.6(L).   Histological image of moderate to marked glandular atrophy in the gastric corpus (×200, H&E). Most of the specialized glands and gastric pits were lost or even disappeared.

epithelium is recognized by the presence of goblet cells, columnar absorptive cells, and the brush border. Endoscopically, areas of intestinal metaplasia may be macroscopically visible as gray–white patches with a slight opalescent tinge and/or a villous appearance. However, the white-light endoscopic features are neither specific enough nor easily found. CLE has been proven to have high accuracy in diagnosing intestinal metaplasia, with a sensitivity of 98.13% and a specificity of 95.33%. In line with histopatholocal findings, the CLE features for intestinal metaplasia are manifested as goblet cells, columnar absorptive cells and the brush border, and villiform foveolar epithelium. Goblet cells in CLE images are large black cells with mucin contrast to surrounding columnar-lined epithelium cells. Columnar absorptive cells and the brush border are more slender, and brighter than columnar mucous cells of normal gastric mucosa, with a clear dark line at the surface of the epithelium. Villiform foveolar epithelium shows a typical villous-like appearance different from the antral or corpus foveolae gastricae (Fig. 9.7).

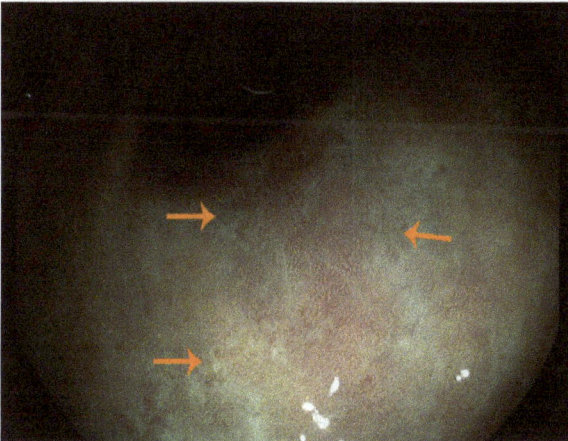

Fig. 9.7(A). High-resolution white-light endoscopy showing intestinal metaplasia in the stomach. IM shows a whitish change with plaques-patches, or homogeneous discoloration on gastric mucosa (*orange arrows*).

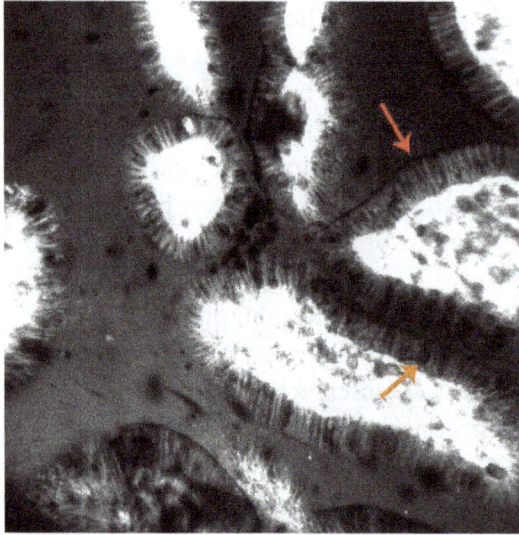

Fig. 9.7(B).   The features of intestinal metaplasia in a CLE image. The typical villous-like appearance (red arrow) and black goblet cells (orange arrow) can be seen (10% fluorescein staining).

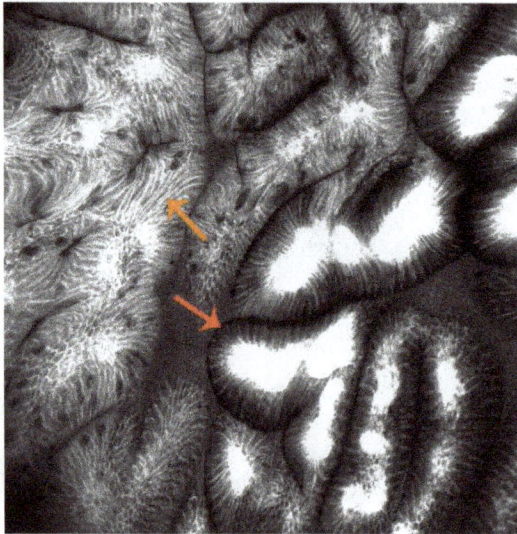

Fig. 9.7(C).   A comparison of IM mucosa (*orange arrow*) and non-IM mucosa (*red arrow*) in an antral CLE image (10% fluorescein staining).

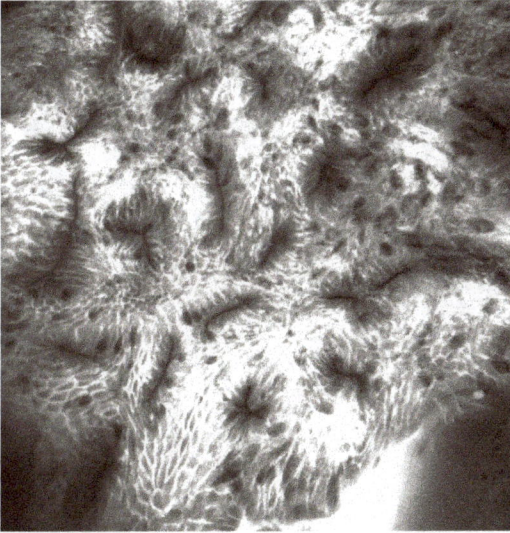

Fig. 9.7(D). Corporal CLE image of intestinal metaplasia (10% fluorescein staining). The dark goblet cells are scattered and the slender and bright epithelial cells can be seen.

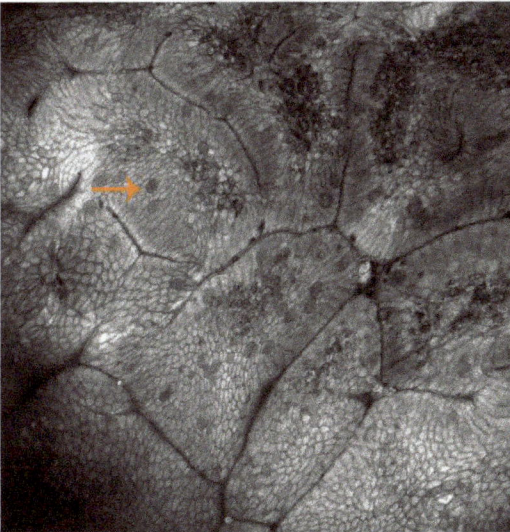

Fig. 9.7(E). Acriflavine-aided endomicroscopy of intestinal metaplasia (0.02% acriflavine staining). The goblet cells can be clearly identified (*orange arrow*).

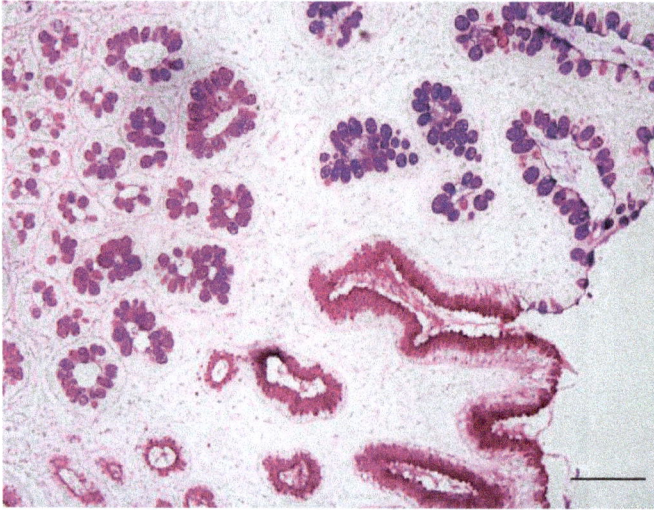

Fig. 9.7(F).　Histochemical stain of intestinal metaplasia (AB/PAS × 400). The blue goblet cells surrounded by nonstaining absorption cells can be seen. The normal columnar epithelial cells filled with acidic and neutral mucus are stained purple.

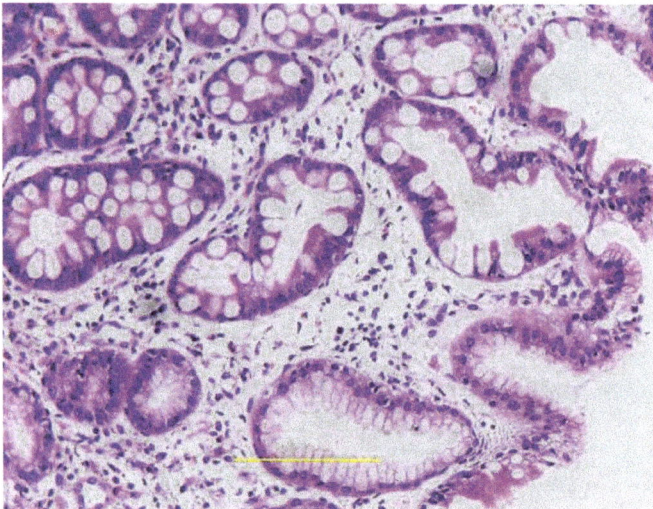

Fig. 9.7(G).　Histochemical image of intestinal metaplasia (×400, H&E). The upper part of the image shows intestinal mucosa, with the villous-like gastric pits and the brush border stained by the eosin color.

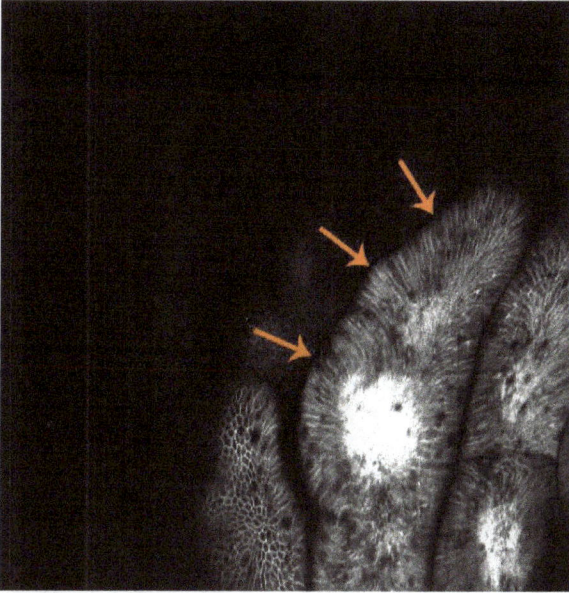

Fig. 9.7(H). The CLE features of the brush border. A black line can be seen around the villous-like gastric pits (*orange arrow*).

Classification of gastric intestinal metaplasia

As with histopathology, intestinal metaplasia can be categorized into complete or incomplete forms by CLE, on the basis of the shape of goblet cells, the presence of absorptive cells or the brush border, and the architecture of vessels and crypts (Figs. 9.8 and 9.9). The CLE features of complete and incomplete intestinal metaplasia are described in Table 9.2.

Severity of gastric intestinal metaplasia

Histological grading of the severity of intestinal metaplasia is according to the visual analog scale of the updated Sydney classification. However, it is based on the area of glandular metaplasia toward a longitudinal section of a specimen. CLE cannot make a similar

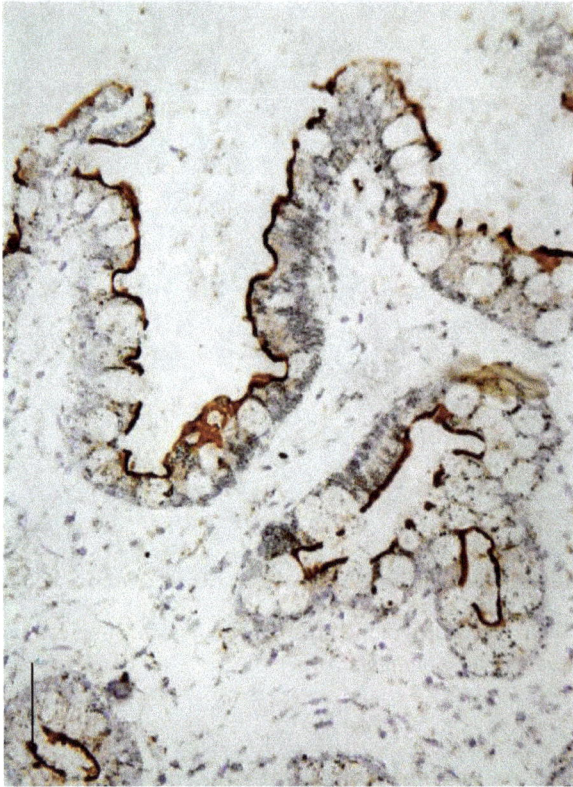

Fig. 9.7(I). CD10 immunohistochemistry image of the brush border (×400, CD10 immunohistochemistry). A clear and neat brown borderline can be seen; it presents the brush border.

Table 9.2. Classification of Gastric Intestinal Metaplasia by CLE[6]

	CLE Features for Intestinal Metaplasia	
	Complete	Incomplete
Goblet cells	Interspersed among absorptive cells with or without brush border	Smaller numbers, scattered among gastric-type cells; without absorptive cells and brush border
Crypts	Regular	Tortuous and branched
Capillaries	Regular	Irregular

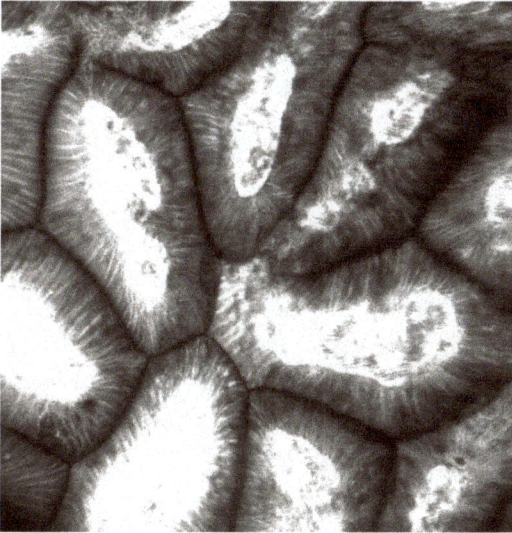

Fig. 9.8(A). CLE image of the complete type of intestinal metaplasia (10% fluorescein staining). Absorptive cells, goblet cells, and the brush border can be identified interspersed among the regular gastric pits and capillaries.

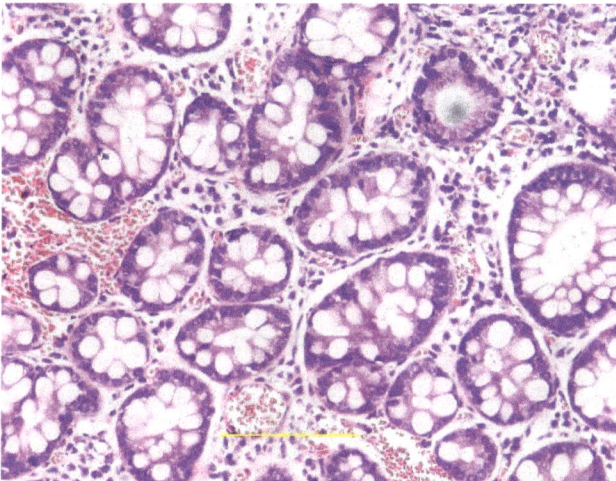

Fig. 9.8(B). Histochemical image of the complete type of intestinal metaplasia (× 400, H&E). Absorptive cells, goblet cells, and the brush border are interspersed among the regular gastric pits and capillaries, which indicates complete intestinal metaplasia.

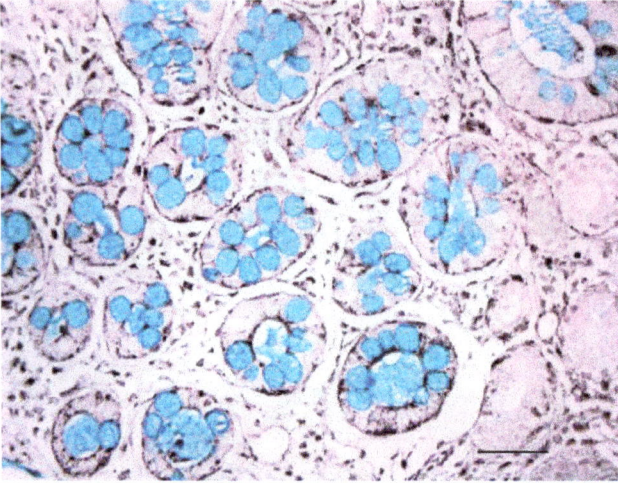

Fig. 9.8(C). Histochemical image of the complete type of intestinal metaplasia (× 400, HID/AB). The goblet cells are stained blue, whereas the columnar epithelial cells are not stained.

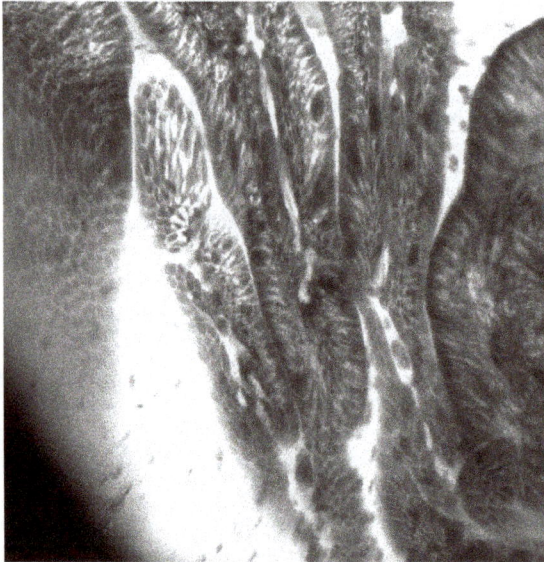

Fig. 9.9(A). CLE image of the incomplete type of intestinal metaplasia (10% fluorescein staining). The villous gastric pits can be seen, with all sizes of goblet cells. The brush border is not clear.

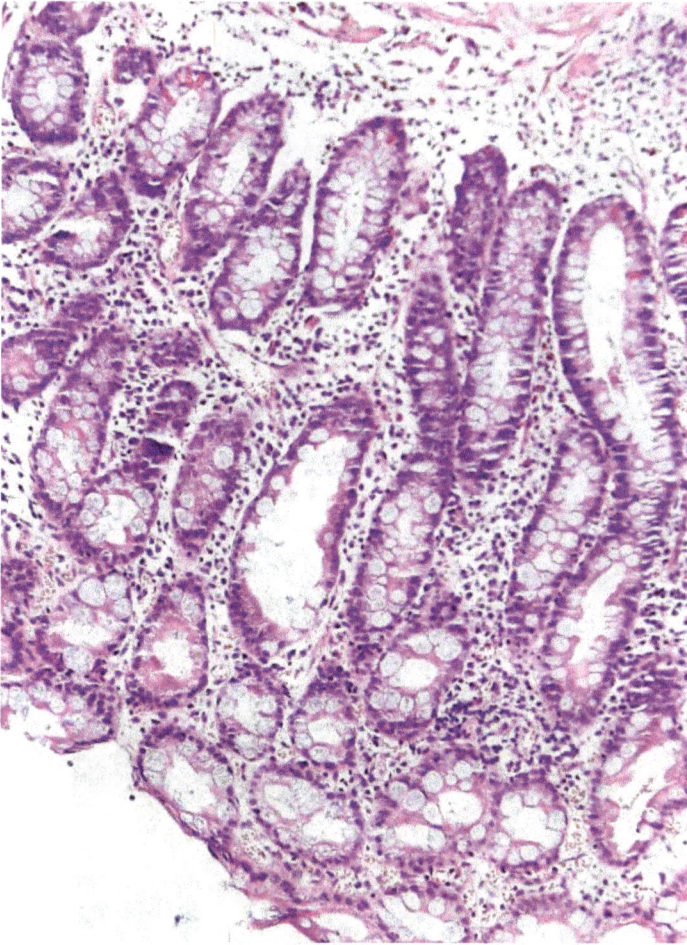

Fig. 9.9(B). Histochemical image of the incomplete type of intestinal metaplasia (× 400, H&E). All sizes of goblet cells can be seen.

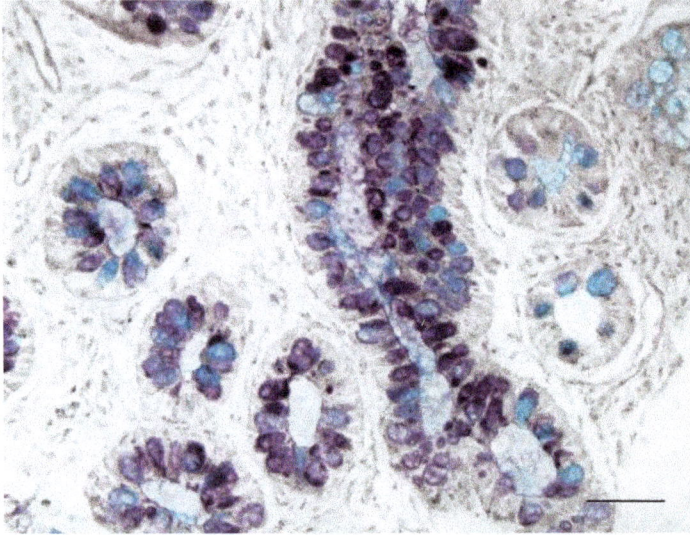

Fig. 9.9(C).   Histochemical image of the incomplete type of intestinal metaplasia (×400, HID/AB). Most of the columnar epithelial cells are stained sepia.

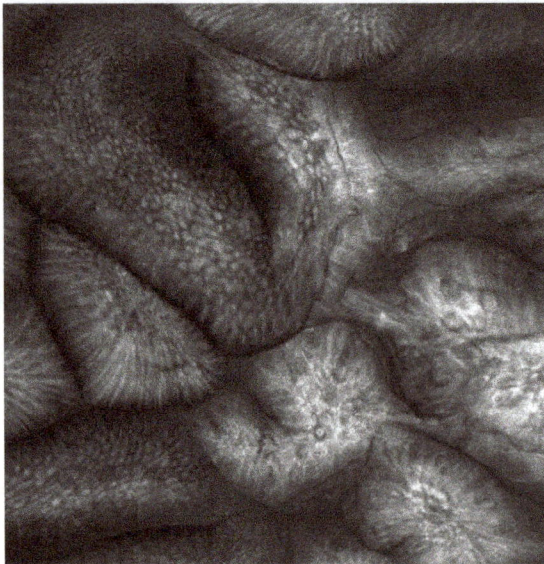

Fig. 9.10(A).   Mild intestinal metaplasia classified by CLE (10% fluorescein staining). The villous glands are distributed uniformly, with less active proliferation.

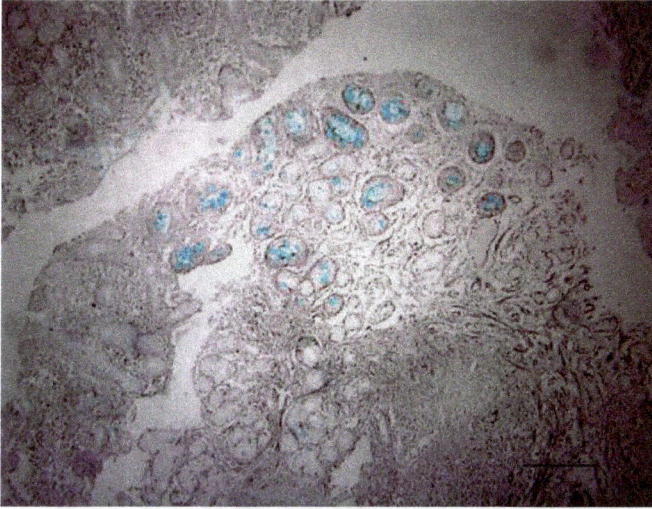

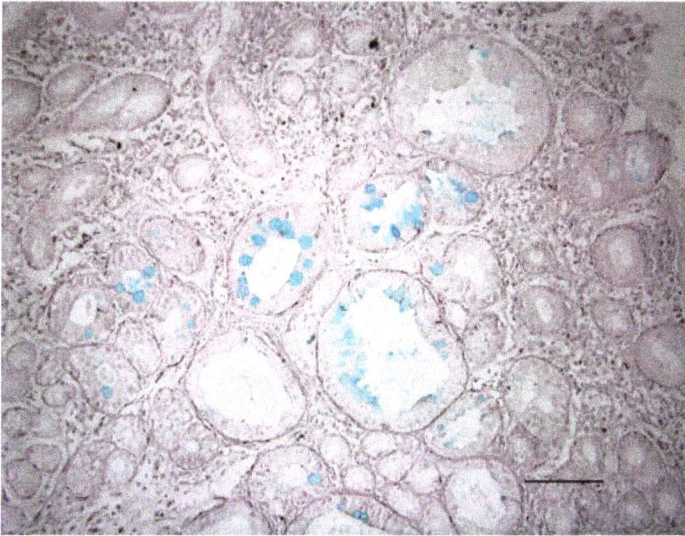

Fig. 9.10(B). Histochemical images of mild intestinal metaplasia (×100, HID/AB, longitudinal section, *top*; ×400, HID/AB, cross-section, *bottom*). Normal gastric glands and small numbers of goblet cells and absorptive epithelial cells can be seen.

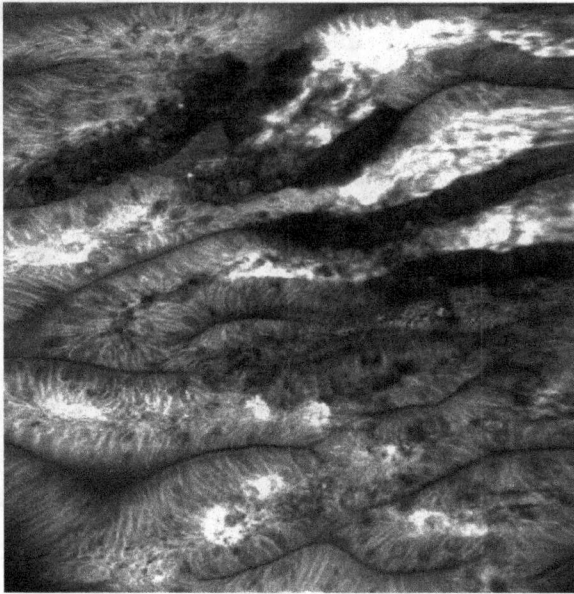

Fig. 9.11(A).   Severe intestinal metaplasia classified by CLE (10% fluorescein staining). The density of the glands is increased and the gland proliferation is active.

grading because of its limited scanning depth (only 0–250 μm). However, various degrees of intestinal metaplasia usually have apparently different features in the shallow mucosal layers. Mild intestinal imetaplasia is usually manifested as uniformly distributed villous glands with less active proliferation, and severe intestinal metaplasia as increased density of intestinal metaplasia glands with active proliferation, which can both be visualized by CLE (Figs. 9.10 and 9.11).

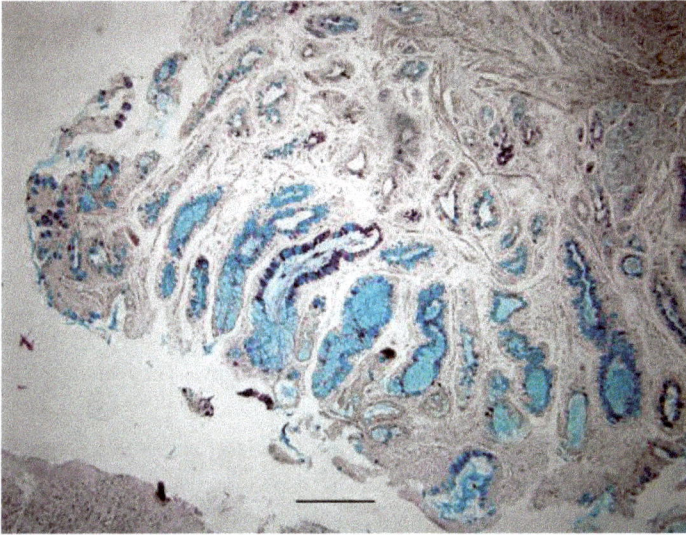

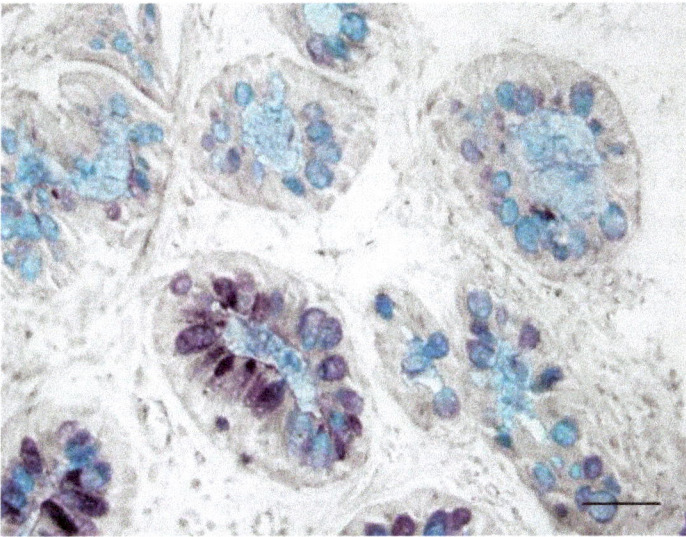

Fig. 9.11(B). Histochemical images of severe intestinal metaplasia (×100, HID/AB, *top*; ×400, HID/AB, *bottom*). Irregularly arranged villous pits and a large quantity of goblet cells can be seen.

References

1. Dixon MF, Genta RM, Yardley JH, *et al.* (1996) Classification and grading of gastritis. The updated Sydney System. International Workshop on the Histopathology of Gastritis, Houston 1994. *Am J Surg Pathol* **20**: 1161–1181.

2. Elta GH, Appelman HD, Behler EM, *et al.* (1987) A study of the correlation between endoscopic and histological diagnoses in gastro-duodenitis. *Am J Gastroenterol* **82**: 749–753.

3. Kiesslich R, Goetz M, Burg J, *et al.* (2005) Diagnosing *Helicobacter pylori in vivo* by confocal laser endoscopy. *Gastroenterology* **128**: 2119–2123.

4. Rui J, YQ L, XM G, *et al.* (2010) Confocal laser endomicroscopy for diagnosis of *Helicobacter pylori* infection: a prospective study. *J Gastroenterol Hepatol* **25**: 700–705.

5. Zhang JN, Li YQ, Zhao YA, *et al.* (2008) Classification of gastric pit patterns by confocal endomicroscopy. *Gastrointest Endosc* **67**: 843–853.

6. Tytgat GN. (1991) The Sydney System: endoscopic division. Endoscopic appearances in gastritis/duodenitis. *J Gastroenterol Hepatol* **6**: 223–234.

7. Guo YT, Li YQ, Yu T, *et al.* (2008) Diagnosis of gastric intestinal metaplasia with confocal laser endomicroscopy *in vivo*: a prospective study. *Endoscopy* **40**: 547–553.

8. Walker MM. (2003) Is intestinal metaplasia of the stomach reversible. *Gut* **52**: 1–4.

Chapter 10

Gastric Intraepithelial Neoplasia

Gastric cancer remains the second-leading cause of cancer-related deaths worldwide, which emphasizes the need for early diagnosis. In terms of geographic distribution, almost two-thirds of gastric cancer occurs in less developed regions. In China, although remarkable declines in gastric cancer mortality have been noticed during the last decade due to the dramatic improvements in the social economy and health service, the absolute number of gastric cancer cases is still a significant burden of the national health program.[1]

According to Correa's model of carcinogenesis, gastric adenocarcinoma, in most instances, represents a multistep process from chronic inflammation, atrophic gastritis, intestinal metaplasia, and intraepithelial neoplasia to carcinoma.[2] Although the biological potential of gastric intraepithelial neoplasia (GIN) as the precursor of gastric carcinoma has been validated, the classification of these lesions was varied between Western and Japanese pathologists until the development of the Vienna classification of gastrointestinal epithelial neoplasia (Table 10.1).[3] A two-tiered system of low- and high-grade GIN is now widely used in all classifications of GIN.

For low grade intraepithelial neoplasia (LGIN), progression to adenocarcinoma was reported in 0%–23% of patients within 1–4 years. Considering the lower rate of malignant transformation of LGIN, annual endoscopic surveillance is recommended and surgical resection is not necessary. In contrast, high grade intraepithelial neoplasia (HGIN) progresses to gastric cancer in 60%–85% of patients over a median interval of 4–48 months.[4] Given the much more ominous outcome of HGIN, endoscopic mucosal resection (EMR) is now widely used in

Table 10.1.   Vienna Classification of Gastrointestinal Epithelial Neoplasia

Category 1	Negative for neoplasia/dysplasia
Category 2	Indefinite for neoplasia/dysplasia
Category 3	Noninvasive low-grade neoplasia
	(low-grade adenoma/dysplasia)
Category 4	Noninvasive high-grade neoplasia
	4.1. High-grade adenoma/dysplasia
	4.2. Noninvasive carcinoma
	(carcinoma *in situ*)
	4.3. Suspicion of invasive carcinoma
Category 5	Invasive neoplasia
	5.1. Intramucosal carcinoma
	5.2. Submucosal carcinoma or beyond

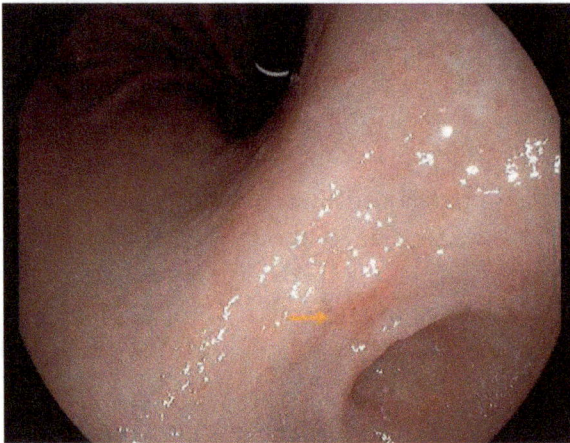

Fig. 10.1.   White-light endoscopy of the stomach shows a superficial flat lesion (IIb) at the gastric angle *(arrow).*

many special centers for definitive therapy of HGIN. Modern endoscopic devices such as chromoendoscopy have improved surveillance of previously unnoticeable mucosal lesions. Furthermore, the diagnostic criteria by magnification chromoendoscopy have been validated for the diagnosis of intestinal metaplasia and dysplasia.[5,6] However, these techniques are limited to the identification of morphological changes of

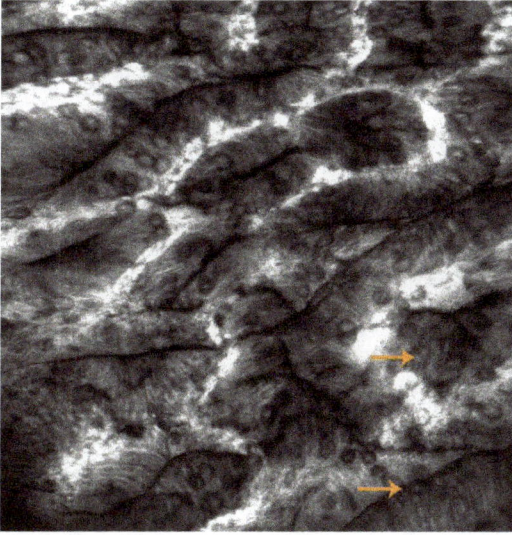

Fig. 10.2. Endomicroscopy of this lesion displays variably sized glands with preserved polarity, mild heterogeneous epithelial heights, and mild stratification of the epithelial cells (*arrows*).

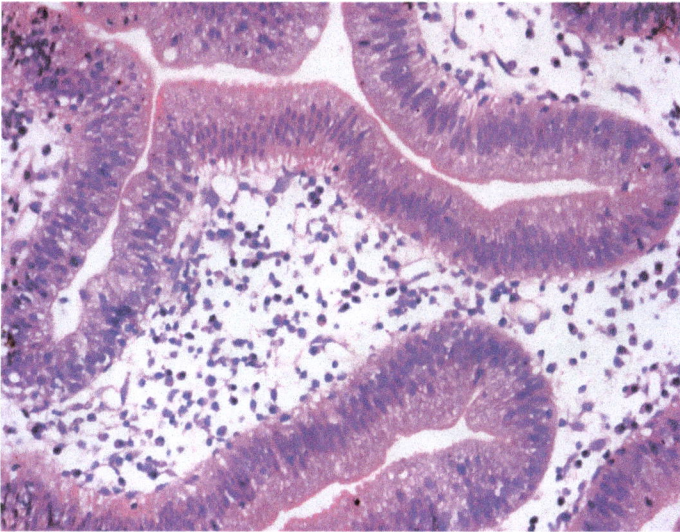

Fig. 10.3. The corresponding histopathology confirmed low grade intraepithelial neoplasia with similar findings in confocal images.

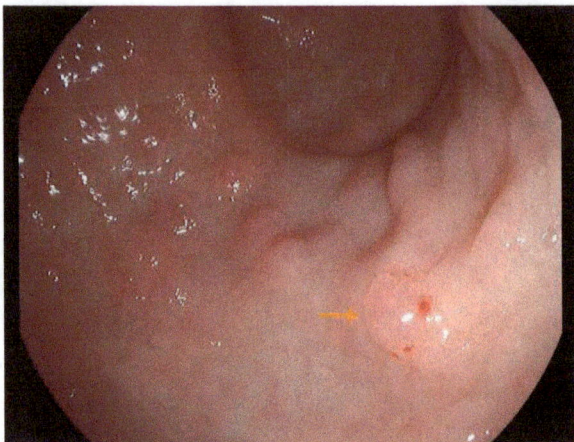

Fig. 10.4. Several sessile polypoid lesions (ls) are displayed by white-light endoscopy, and a suspected lesion is identified during endomicroscopy (*arrow*).

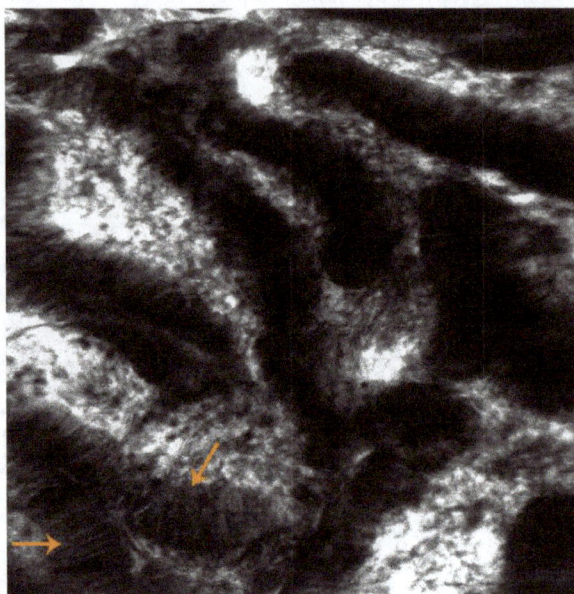

Fig. 10.5. Sequential endomicroscopic imaging of the suspected lesion shows mild to moderate irregularity of the glandular arrangement, mild unevenness of the epithelium, and mild elongation of the epithelial cells (*arrows*).

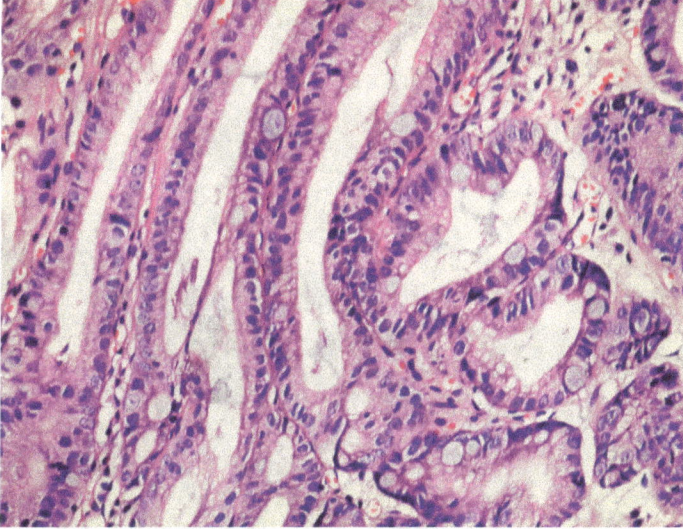

Fig. 10.6. Histopathology of the targeted biopsy specimen shows low grade intraepithelial neoplasia.

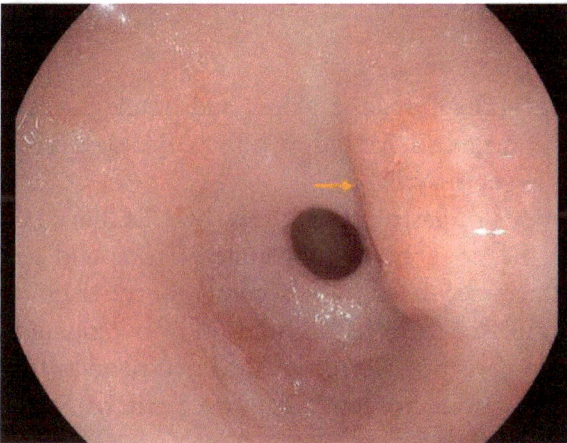

Fig. 10.7. A 1.5 × 2.0 cm elevated lesion at the posterior wall of the antrum is recognized by white-light endoscopy (*arrow*).

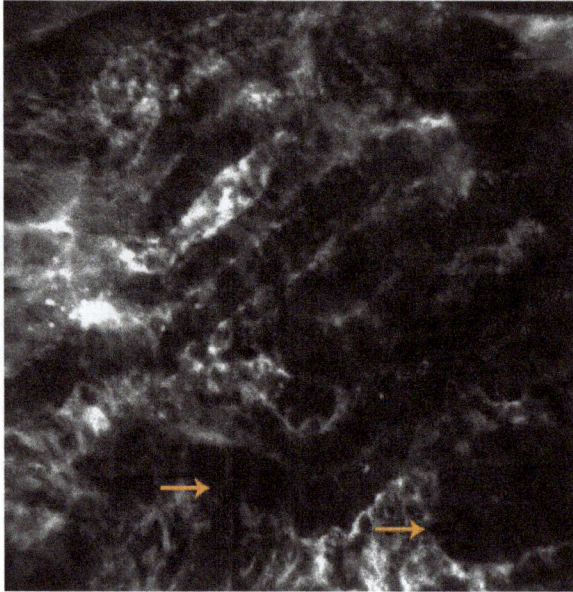

Fig. 10.8.   Endomicroscopy shows highly irregular glands with loss of polarity, obvious epithelial thickness, and severely stratified epithelial cells (*arrows*) with increased density.

gastric mucosa, and still require biopsy and histological assessment for confirmation of diagnosis. Moreover, endoscopic classification of LGIN and HGIN is as yet unavailable.

Classifications of gastric pit patterns by CLE have been found to be useful for the prediction of atrophic gastritis and gastric cancer, and CLE has been validated to be accurate for the diagnosis of gastric intestinal metaplasia *in vivo.*[7,8] Studies also investigated the usefulness of CLE in detecting Barrett's associated neoplasia.[9,10] However, clearly defined endomicroscopic diagnostic criteria for GIN are still lacking.

According to the histological diagnostic criteria for GIN, the intraepithelial neoplastic gastric epithelium should have the following features: (1) increased proliferation of the cells; (2) abnormal morphology and pleomorphism of the cells; (3) architectural derangement of glands; (4) stromal changes.[11] As in the case with histological features, distinctive abnormalities on gland architecture, cell morphology, and vessel architecture in CLE images can be identified in GIN lesions. The following images shows clinical examples of GIN.

References

1. Yang L. (2006) Incidence and mortality of gastric cancer in China. *World J Gastroenterol* **12**: 17–20.
2. Correa P. (1992) Human gastric carcinogenesis: a multistep and multifactorial process — First American Cancer Society Award Lecture on Cancer Epidemiology and Prevention. *Cancer Res* **52**: 6735–6740.
3. Schlemper RJ, Riddell RH, Kato Y, *et al.* (2000) The Vienna classification of gastrointestinal epithelial neoplasia. *Gut* **47**: 251–255.
4. Yamada H, Ikegami M, Shimoda T, *et al.* (2004) Long-term follow-up study of gastric adenoma/dysplasia. *Endoscopy* **36**: 390–396.
5. Dinis-Ribeiro M, da Costa-Pereira A, Lopes C, *et al.* (2003) Magnification chromoendoscopy for the diagnosis of gastric intestinal metaplasia and dysplasia. *Gastrointest Endosc* **57**: 498–504.
6. Areia M, Amaro P, Dinis-Ribeiro M, *et al.* (2008) External validation of a classification for methylene blue magnification chromoendoscopy in premalignant gastric lesions. *Gastrointest Endosc* **67**: 1011–1018.
7. Zhang JN, Li YQ, Zhao YA, *et al.* (2008) Classification of gastric pit patterns by confocal endomicroscopy. *Gastrointest Endosc* **67**: 843–853.
8. Guo YT, Li YQ, Yu T, *et al.* (2008) Diagnosis of gastric intestinal metaplasia with confocal laser endomicroscopy *in vivo*: a prospective study. *Endoscopy* **40**: 547–553.
9. Kiesslich R, Gossner L, Goetz M, *et al.* (2006) *In vivo* histology of Barrett's esophagus and associated neoplasia by confocal laser endomicroscopy. *Clin Gastroenterol Hepatol* **4**: 979–987.
10. Dunbar KB, Okolo P, 3rd, Montgomery E, Canto MI. (2009) Confocal laser endomicroscopy in Barrett's esophagus and endoscopically inapparent Barrett's neoplasia: a prospective, randomized, double-blind, controlled, crossover trial. *Gastrointest Endosc* **70**: 645–654.
11. Ming SC, Bajtai A, Correa P, *et al.* (1984) Gastric dysplasia: significance and pathologic criteria. *Cancer* **54**: 1794–1801.

Chapter 11

Gastric Tumor

Gastric tumor is subdivided into two main categories: benign and malignant. Because CLE has a scanning depth of 0–250 μm, this section deals only with gastric epithelial tumors. Benign epithelial tumors are known as adenomas, and malignant epithelial tumors are composed of adenocarcinoma and other variants of carcinoma. So, mainly adenoma and adenocarcinoma are discussed.

Gastric Adenoma

Gastric adenomas, defined as lesions composed of tubules or villi of dysplastic epithelium, are largely accepted as a premalignant condition in the stomach. According to the WHO classification,[1] gastric adenomas can be classified into tubular, villous, and tubulovillous adenomas, and two subtypes of low-grade or high-grade adenoma can be further classified according to the revised Vienna classification.[2]

There are specific features of gastric adenoma in both fluorescein- and acriflavine-aided CLE images (Figs. 11.1 and 11.2). When 10% fluorescein sodium is applied intravenously, CLE images for adenomas show a distinct cell type with a tessellated appearance identified as an "atypical cell." The atypical cell is manifested as a type of black cell of irregular shape encircled with white interstices. After 0.02% acriflavine is applied topically, atypical cells can be recognized as high gray-scale cells with irregular shape, nonuniform size, and enlarged nuclei. Moreover, gastric adenomas, whether tubular or villous, show significant architectural changes. Irregular ridges or villi, which sometimes have a "cerebriform" shape, are usually observed. Focal asymmetrical

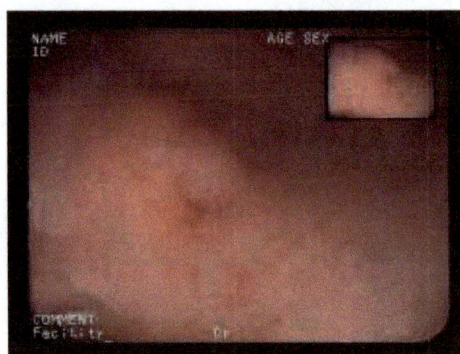

Fig. 11.1. Endoscopic, histologic, and CLE image of a gastric adenoma. **(A)** Conventional white-light endoscopic view.

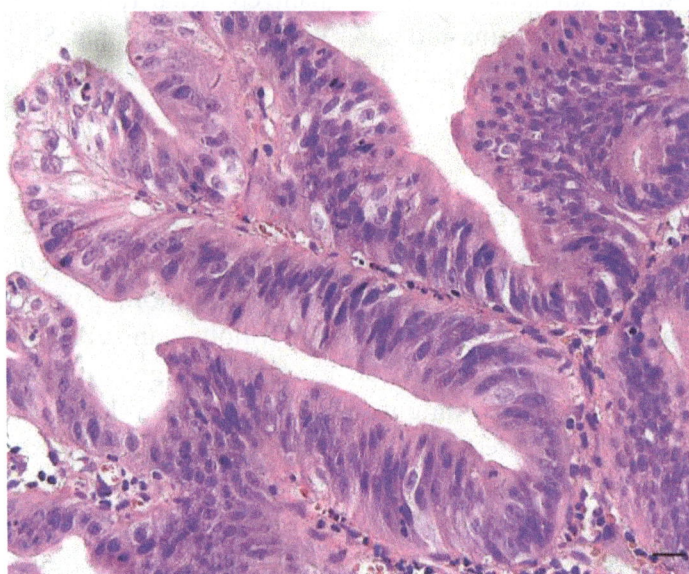

Fig. 11.1(B). The corresponding histologic specimen shows a tubulovillous adenoma (H&E, original magnification × 400).

ridge distortion is also often seen, implying the presence of dysplasia. Lip-shaped or ridgelike openings of glands in different lengths and widths are often observed when tubular components predominate. In addition, another cell type, with a light-gray appearance similar to an

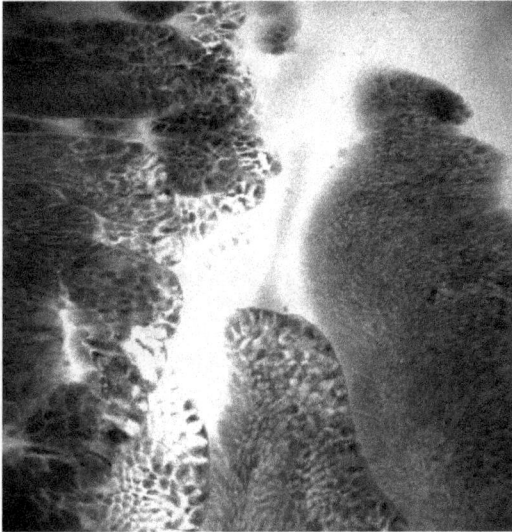

Fig. 11.1(C). Fluorescein-aided CLE imaging of the adenoma: black cells of irregular shape encircled with white interstices.

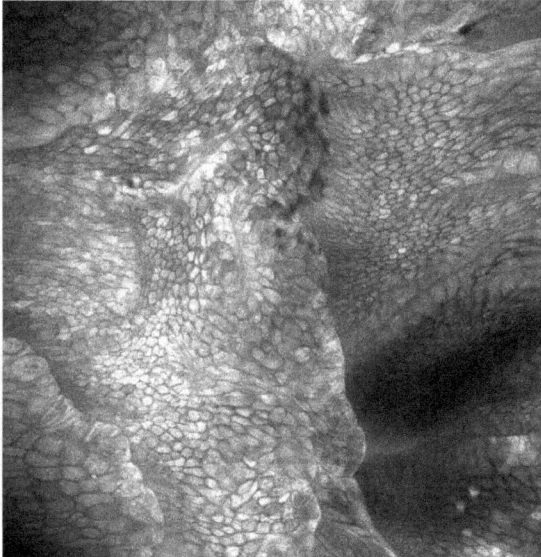

Fig. 11.1(D). Acriflavine-aided CLE imaging of the adenoma: high gray-scale cells with irregular size and enlarged nuclei. Focal asymmetrical ridge distortion and atypical cells are observed.

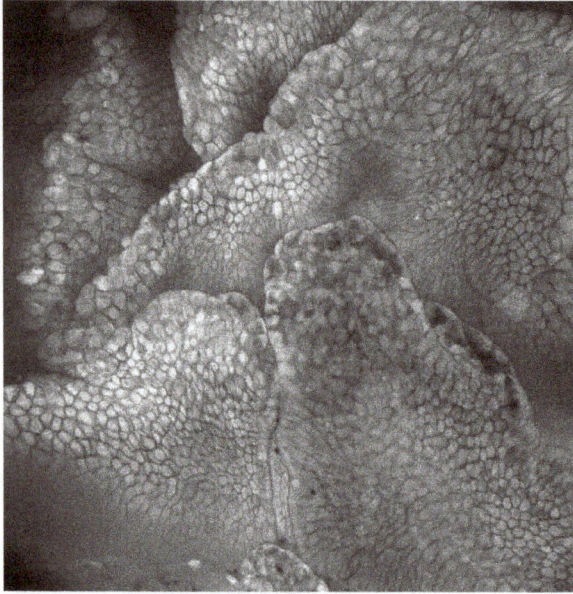

Fig. 11.1(E).   The cerebriform shape and the openings of tubular glands.

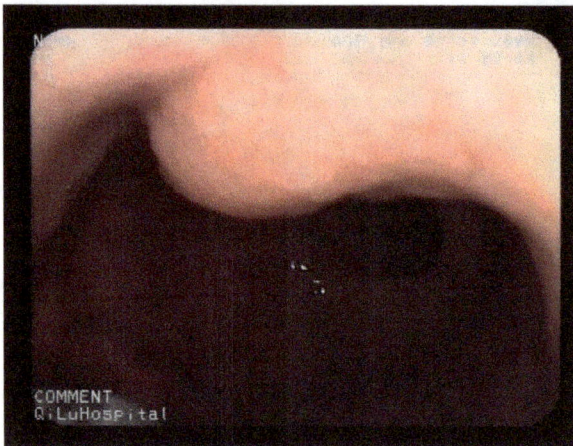

Fig. 11.2.   Endoscopic, histologic, and confocal images of a gastric adenoma. **(A)** Conventional white-light endoscopic view.

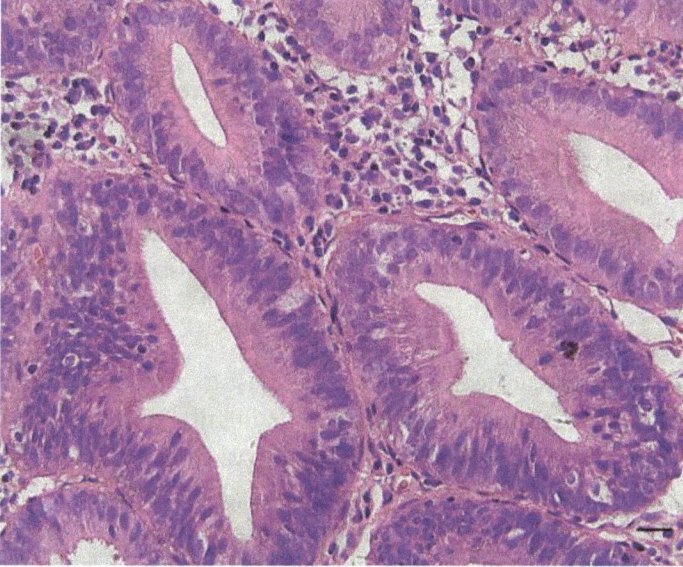

Fig. 11.2(B). The corresponding histologic specimen shows a tubular adenoma (H&E, original magnification × 400).

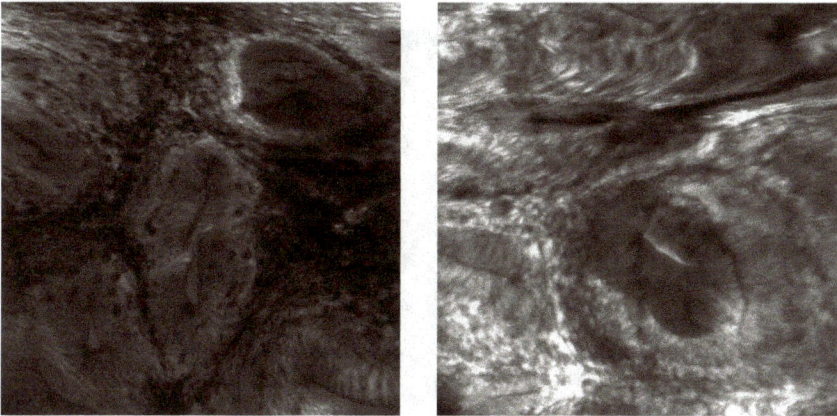

Fig. 11.2(C). Fluorescein-aided CLE imaging of the adenoma. Tubular glands are composed of atypical cells.

"absorptive cell," is also seen; it is more slender than the normal gastric columnar epithelium cell.

Gastric adenomas are sometimes easily confused with gastric hyperplastic polyps during conventional endoscopy. Hyperplastic polyps have less malignant potential (1.5%–3%), but adenomas have an incidence of malignant transformation ranging from 4% to 70%.[3,4] Therefore, adenomas should be distinguished accurately from hyperplastic polyps. Superior to conventional endoscopy, CLE has the ability to identify the histological features of hyperplastic polyps and adenomas (Figs. 11.1 and 11.4).

The histological feature of hyperplastic polyps is prolonged, branching, and serrated crypts with cystic dilation and the lamina propria with significant edema and inflammation infiltration. In CLE images, marked hyperplasia of surface epithelial cells covers the gastric pits nearest the lumen, with a normal feature identical to the surrounding epithelial cells with no atypia. In addition, the prolonging and enlarging of the gastric pits lead to a decreased number of pits during a single visual field.

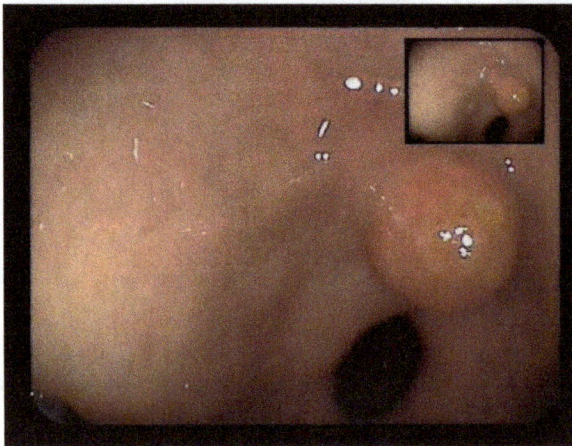

Fig. 11.3.   Endoscopic, histologic, and confocal images of a gastric hyperplastic polyp. **(A)** Conventional white-light endoscopic view of an antral semipedunculated polyp.

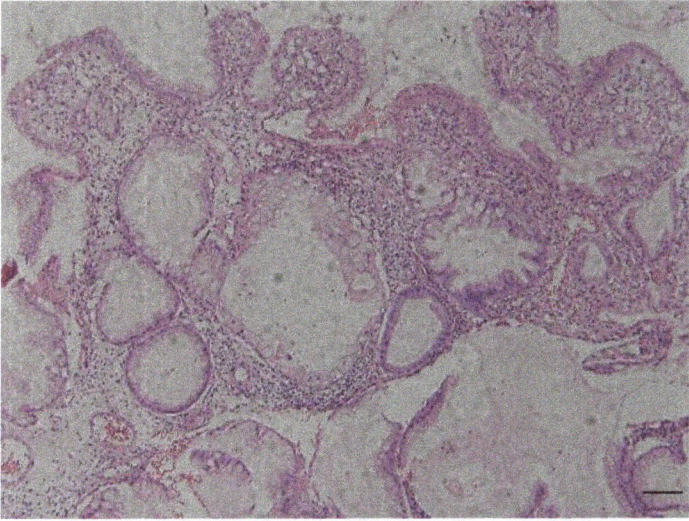

Fig. 11.3(B). The corresponding histological specimen shows a hyperplastic polyp (H&E, original magnification × 100).

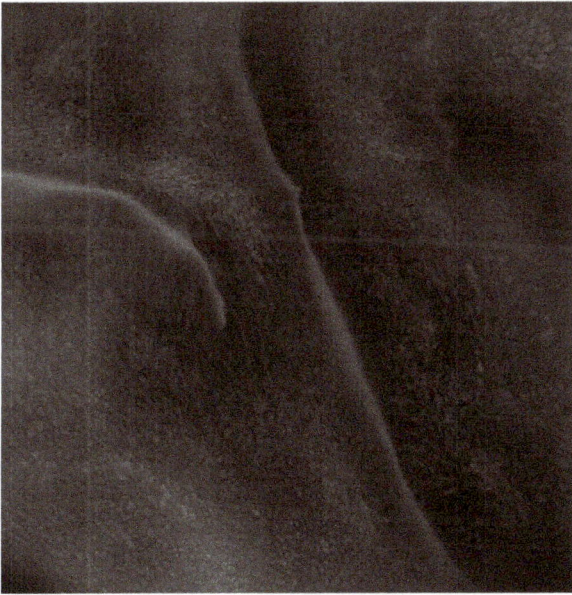

Fig. 11.3(C). CLE images after fluorescein injection. Surface confocal image of the polyp. Marked hyperplasia of surface columnar epithelium cells without any atypia.

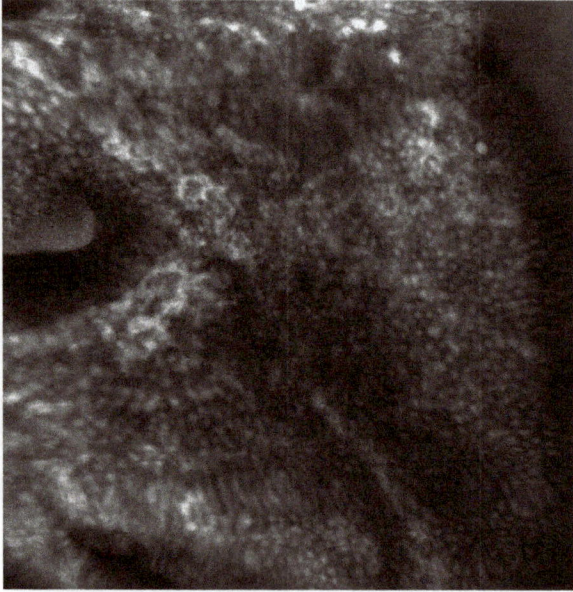

Fig. 11.3(D).   Edematous mucosa and inflammatory cells.

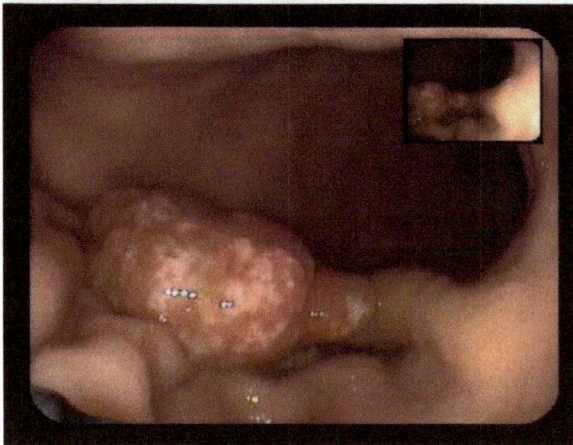

Fig. 11.4.   Endoscopic, histologic, and confocal images of a gastric hyperplastic polyp. **(A)** Conventional white-light endoscopic view of a pedunculated polyp in the gastric body.

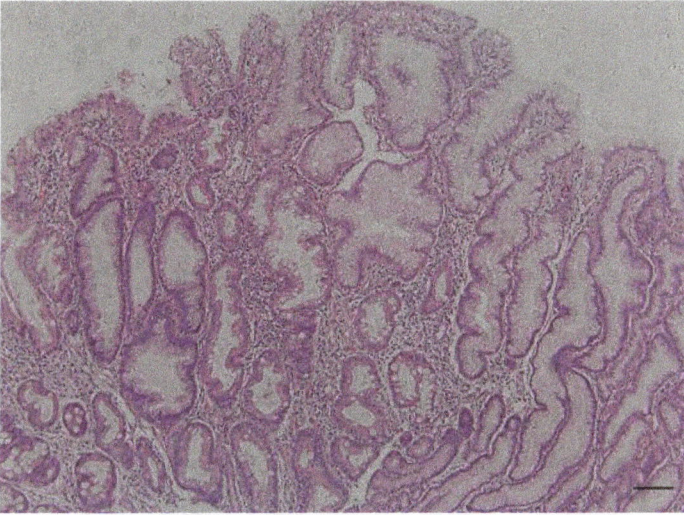

Fig. 11.4(B). The corresponding histologic specimen shows a hyperplastic polyp (H&E, original magnification × 100).

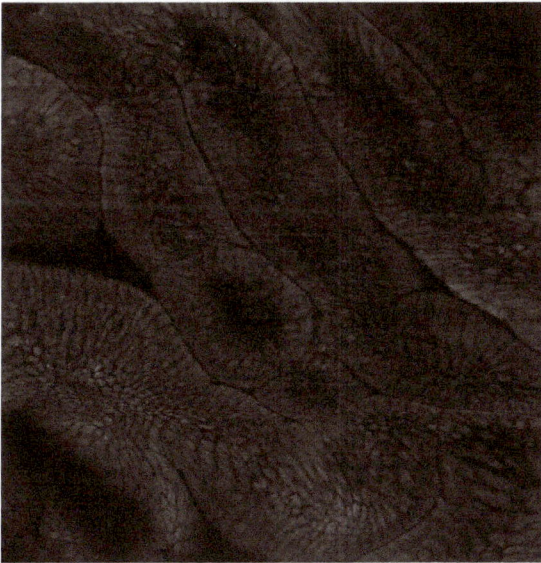

Fig. 11.4(C). CLE images of the polyp after fluorescein injection or topical acri-flavine.

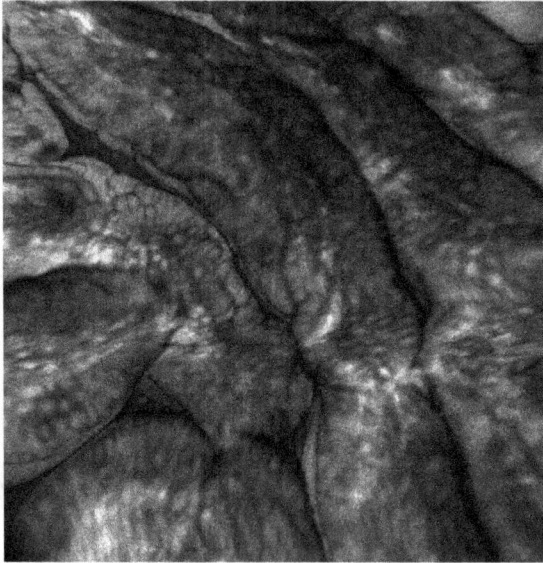

Fig. 11.4(D). Markedly hyperplastic gastric columnar epithelial cells and elongated or branchlike gastric pits.

The CLE imaging criteria for gastric hyperplastic polyps and adenomas are summarized in Table 11.1. In our study with 60 gastric hyperplastic polyps and 27 gastric adenomas,[5] *in vivo* CLE differential diagnosis was made as compared with the histological findings. The overall accuracy of *in vivo* CLE diagnosis was 90% [95% confidence interval (CI): 83%–96%], and the kappa coefficient of agreement between histopathology and *in vivo* CLE imaging was 0.77. CLE differential diagnosis after endoscopy was made, too. The overall accuracy was 97% (95% CI: 90%–99%), and the kappa coefficient of agreement between histopathology and CLE diagnosis was 0.92. Intraobserver agreement was almost perfect ($\kappa = 0.92$; 95% CI: 0.82–0.99), and interobserver agreement was also excellent ($\kappa = 0.83$; 95% CI: 0.70–0.96).

Gastric Adenocarcinoma

Gastric carcinoma is one of the leading causes of cancer death throughout the world. Several histological classifications have been

Table 11.1. CLE Imaging Criteria for Gastric Hyperplastic Polyps and Adenomas

	Hyperplastic Polyps	Adenomas
Cytological feature	Regular columnar epithelium cells with a megagon shape covering gastric pits; identical to normal surface columnar epithelium cells.	Black cells of irregular shape encircled with white interstices after intravenous fluorescein; high gray-scale cells with irregular size and enlarged nuclei after topical acriflavine.
Crypt architecture	Hyperplastic columnar epithelium cells regularly arranged and encircling the openings of elongated or branch-like pits; dilated, distorted foveolar sulci.	Irregular ridges or villi with a cerebriform shape; focal asymmetrical ridge distortion after topical acriflavine; long ridge-like openings of glands.

proposed, and the WHO classification and Lauren classification are currently widely used. The overwhelming majority of gastric carcinomas are adenocarcinomas.

Early gastric cancer (EGC) is defined as a carcinoma which is limited to the mucosa, or the mucosa and submucosa, irrespective of whether or not metastasis to lymph nodes has occurred.[6] On the basis of macroscopic appearances, EGCs can be classified into three main types (I, II, and III) and three subtypes (IIa, IIb, and IIc).[6,7] The histologic classifications of EGC are similar to those of advanced carcinoma. In the WHO classification, most cases are tubular or signet ring cell in type. In the Lauren classification, most are intestinal carcinomas and one-third are diffuse.

Recently, CLE has shown its value for gastric carcinomas.[8–10] The distinction is based on irregular and abnormal signs of architecture, cells, or microvessels on CLE images (Figs. 11.5–11.8). Abnormal architecture is characterized by loss of regular surface patterns and appearance of atypical glands or disorganized patterns; atypical cells are often dark, irregular in shape and size, and disordered; abnormal microvessels are rigid or irregular, with an increased caliber and an

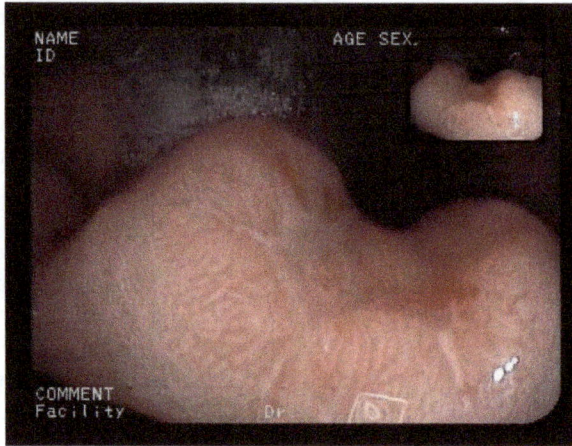

Fig. 11.5. Endoscopic, histologic, and confocal images of an early gastric cancer. **(A)** Conventional white-light endoscopic view of a Paris 0-1 lesion in the gastric body.

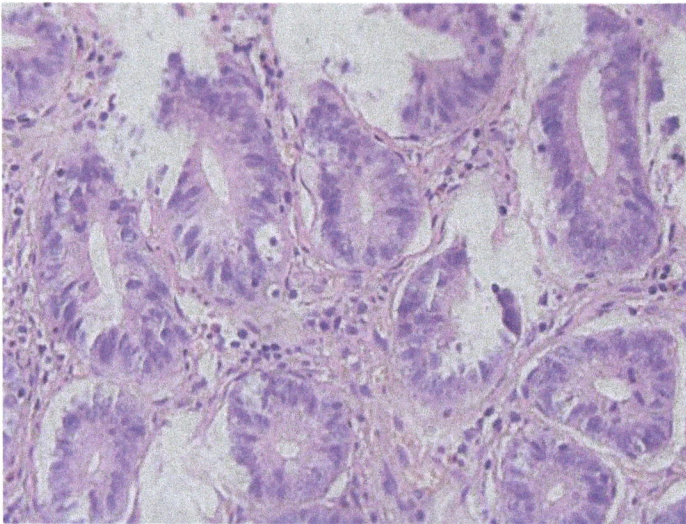

Fig. 11.5(B). The corresponding histologic specimen shows a well-differentiated adenocarcinoma (H&E, original magnification × 400).

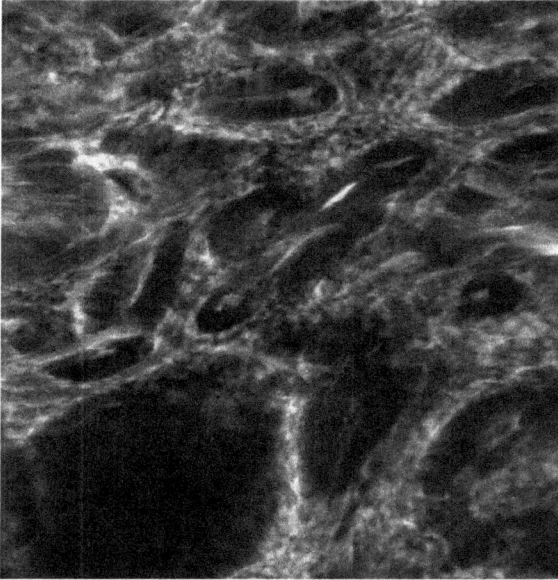

Fig. 11.5(C). CLE images after fluorescein injection. Black column-like cells arranged irregularly and a reduced number of goblet cells.

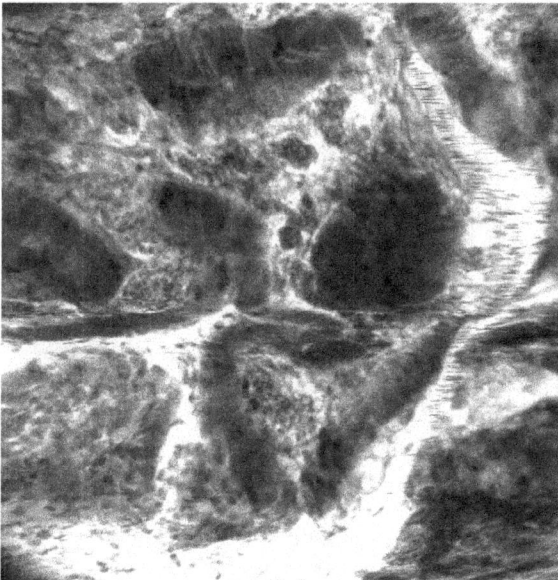

Fig. 11.5(D). Tubular atypical glands with abnormal microvessels.

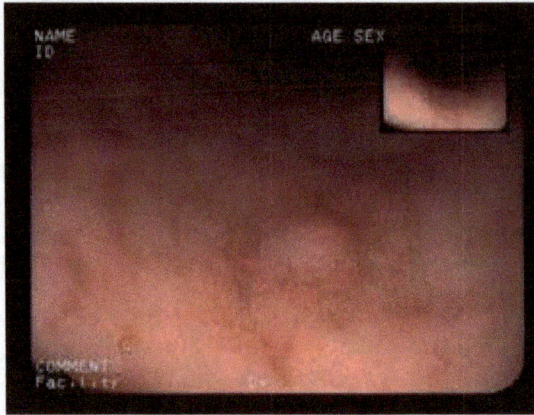

Fig. 11.6.   Endoscopic, histologic, and confocal images of an early gastric cancer. **(A)** Conventional white-light endoscopic view of a Paris 0-IIc + IIa lesion in the gastric body.

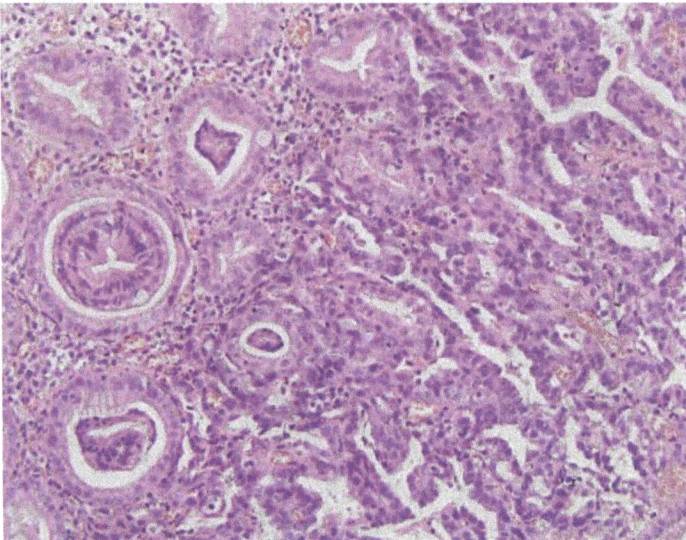

Fig. 11.6(B).   The corresponding histologic specimen shows a moderately differentiated adenocarcinoma (H&E, original magnification × 400).

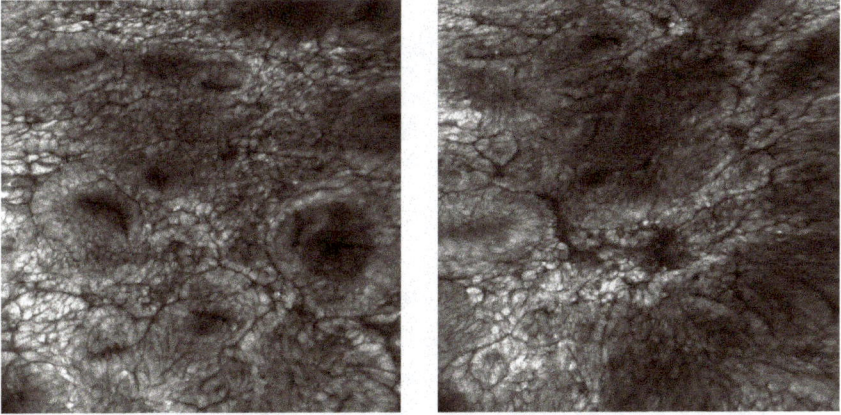

Fig. 11.6(C). CLE images after topical acriflavine: disarranged structure and irregular nuclei.

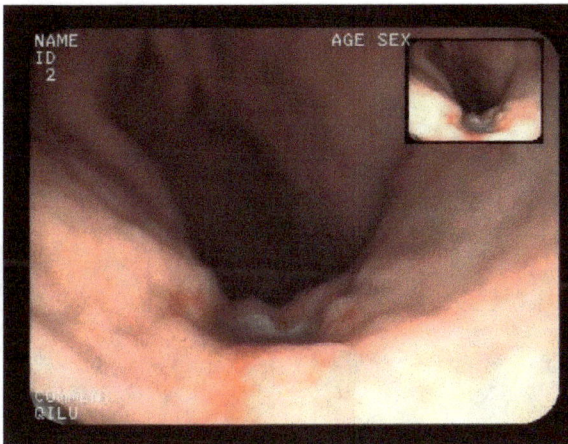

Fig. 11.7. Endoscopic, histologic, and confocal images of an early gastric cancer. **(A)** Conventional white-light endoscopic view of a Paris 0-III lesion in the gastric body.

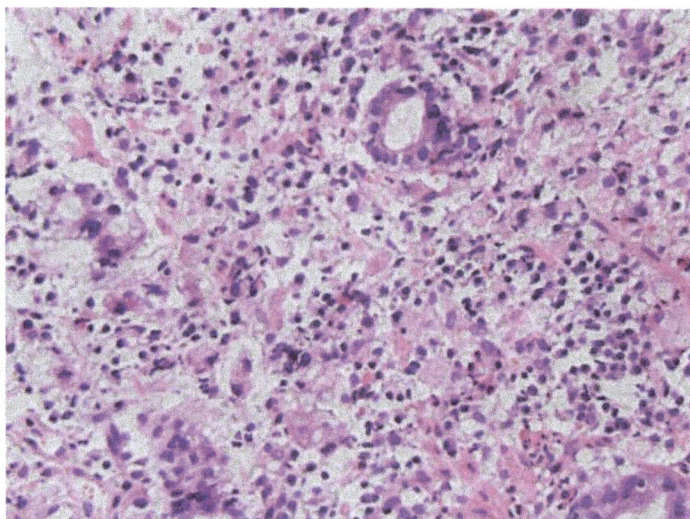

Fig. 11.7(B).   The corresponding histologic specimen shows a poorly differentiated adenocarcinoma (H&E, original magnification × 400).

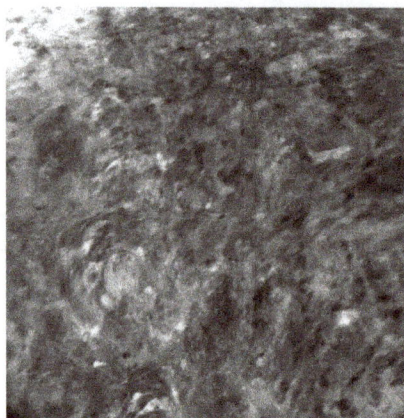

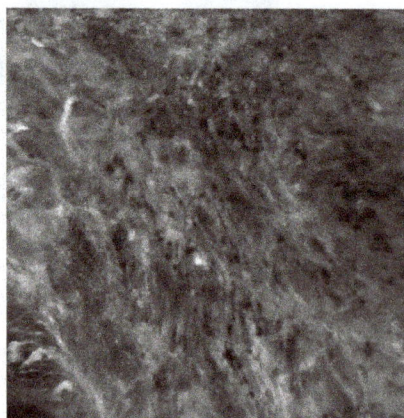

Fig. 11.7(C).   CLE images after fluorescein injection: irregular black cells with poorly formed glands and irregular short-branched microvessels.

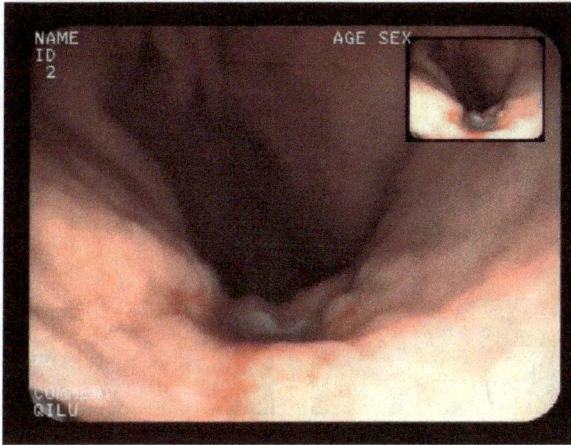

Fig. 11.8. Endoscopic, histologic, and confocal images of an early gastric cancer. **(A)** Conventional white-light endoscopic view of a Paris 0-IIa + IIc lesion in the gastric body.

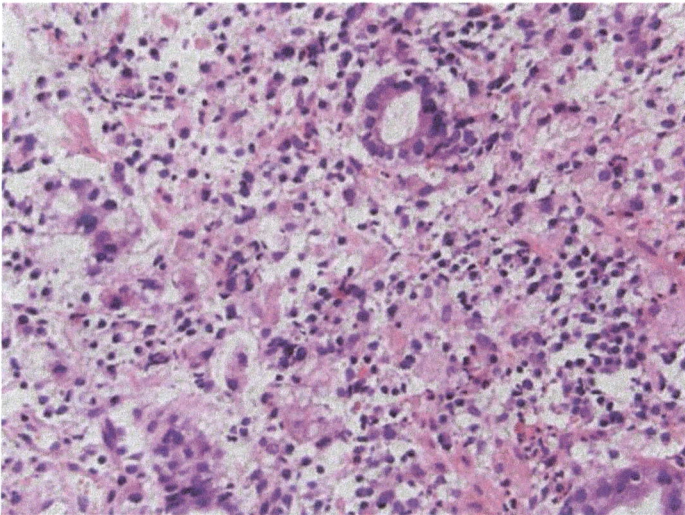

Fig. 11.8(B). The corresponding histologic specimen shows a signet ring cell carcinoma (H&E, original magnification ×400).

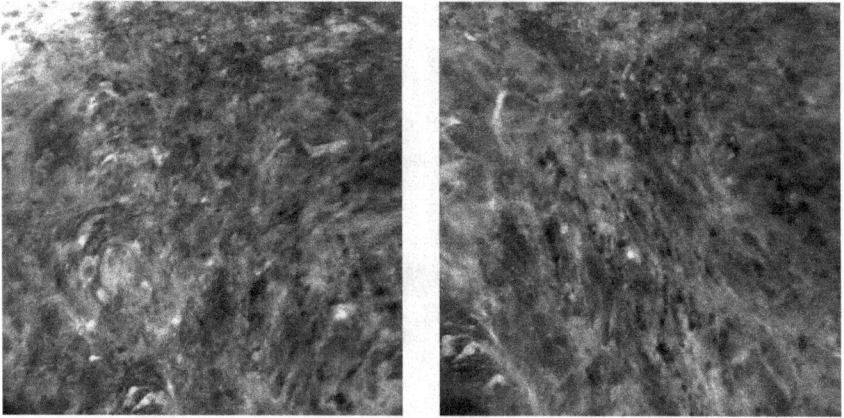

Fig. 11.8(C).   CLE images after fluorescein injection: irregular cells and microvessels with poorly formed glands.

unusual shape. The CLE imaging criteria for gastric mucosal lesions are summarized in Table 11.2.

Kakeji *et al.* examined *ex vivo* normal and malignant tissues of 27 gastric cancers using CLE,[8] and Kitabatake *et al.* obtained *in vivo* CLE images from normal mucosa and cancerous lesions in 27 patients with EGC.[9] These preliminary results showed that gastric cancer could be differentiated from normal mucosa by CLE with a sensitivity of 81.8%–92.6%, a specificity of 97.6%–100%, and an accuracy of 94.2%–96.3%, as compared with histologic findings. Gastric carcinoma is believed to arise from a series of premalignant lesions: atrophic gastritis, IM, and dysplasia. Numerous studies have also demonstrated that gastric cancerous lesions are found in association with a number of different noncancerous lesions. Then, our studies with 182 patients [EGC, 42; high-grade intraepithelial neoplasia (HGIN), 9; low-grade intraepithelial neoplasia (LGIN), 30; intestinal metaplasia (IM); and chronic gastritis, 52] showed that gastric adenocarcinomas could be determined by CLE with a high sensitivity (88.1%) and specificity (98.6%); and gastric neoplastic lesions [adenocarcinoma + intraepithelial neoplasia (IN)] could be identified by CLE with 84.0% sensitivity and 92.1% specificity; however, gastric

Table 11.2. CLE Imaging Criteria for Superficial Gastric Mucosal Lesions

	Architecture	Cells	Microvessels
Not IM, not IN	Surface patterns of gastric types.	Regular, orderly columnar cells; normality of cell polarity.	Normal caliber and shape; regular.
IM	Villous appearance.	Large, black "goblet cells"; slender, tall, bright "absorptive" cells.	Normal caliber and shape; regular.
IN	Glands heterogeneous in shape and size; heterogeneous epithelial thickness; preserved glands.	Increase in epithelial stratification; abnormality of cell polarity.	Normal shape and regular.
Cancer	Loss of regular pit patterns; disorganized or destroyed.	Irregular and disordered cells.	Increased caliber and irregular.

IM — intestinal metaplasia; IN — intraepithelial neoplasia.

intraepithelial neoplasias (GINs) were recognized by CLE with a low sensitivity (66.7%) and high specificity (92.3%).

As shown in our and other previous published studies, the characteristics of CLE images vary by diseases — inflammation, IM, IN, or cancer. However, the distinction between LGIN and gastritis was still unsatisfactory; HGIN was easily confused with cancer; and well-differentiated adenocarcinoma was also sometimes misdiagnosed as IM by CLE. Therefore, we proposed a simple CLE classification for gastric mucosal lesions: noncancerous lesions, and cancer or suspected cancer lesions (Table 11.3). The former was benign and composed of LGIN and other benign lesions, and the latter, involving HGIN and cancer, was regarded as malignant. This proposal was based on several reasons. First, the repeatability or reproducibility of CLE diagnosis for gastric mucosal lesions would be nice. The distinction between LGIN

Table 11.3. Two-tiered CLE System for Determining Gastric Mucosal Lesions

Feature	Noncancerous Lesions	Cancer or Suspected Cancer
Architecture	Regular or mildly heterogeneous.	Obviously heterogeneous; severely disorganized or destroyed.
Cells	Regular or mildly unusual; normality of cell polarity.	Irregular or atypical cells; severe stratification; loss of cell polarity.
Microvessels	Normal caliber and shape, and regular.	Irregular in shape and caliber.

and inflammation is especially difficult and the reported interobserver variation in the diagnosis of LGIN is large.[2] As well, HGIN is recognized more reproducibly, but HGIN does not differ much from cancer, and cancer is often underdiagnosed as HGIN on biopsy.[2,11,12] Second, this proposal could provide meaningful risk stratification and management guidelines. LGIN lesions seldom progress to cancer, but HGIN lesions readily evolve to cancer.[11,12] Lesions with HGIN or cancer are often recommended for resection, whereas follow-up is usually recommended for nonneoplastic or LGIN lesions.[2]

According to the two-tiered CLE system, cancer or suspected cancer lesions could be distinguished from noncancerous lesions by CLE with a high sensitivity (90.2%; 95% CI: 82.0%–98.4%), specificity (98.5%; 94.6%–99.8%), PPV (95.8%; 85.7%–99.55%), NPV (96.3%; 93.1%–99.5%), and accuracy (96.2%; 93.4%–98.9%). Intra- and interobserver agreement was 0.827 (95% CI: 0.759–0.891) and 0.783 (95% CI: 0.712–0.874), respectively, for differentiating benign and malignant lesions.

References

1. Hamilton SR, Aaltonen LA, eds. (2000) *World Health Organization Classification of Tumors: Pathology and Genetics of Tumors of the Digestive System.* International Agency for Research on Cancer (IARC) Press, Lyon, pp. 38–52.

2. Stolte M. (2003) The new Vienna classification of epithelial neoplasia of the gastrointestinal tract: advantages and disadvantages. *Virchows Arch* **442**: 99–106.

3. Orlowska J, Jarosz D, Pachlewski J, Butruk E. (1995) Malignant transformation of benign epithelial gastric polyps. *Am J Gastroenterol* **90**: 2152–2159.

4. Cristallini E, Ascani S, Bolis G. (1992) Association between histologic type of polyp and carcinoma in the stomach. *Gastrointest Endosc* **38**: 481–484.

5. Li WB, Zuo XL, Zuo F, *et al.* (2010) Characterization and identification of gastric hyperplastic polyps and adenomas by confocal laser endomicroscopy. *Surg Endosc* **24**: 517–524.

6. Japanese Gastric Cancer Association. (1998) *Japanese classification of gastric carcinoma,* 2nd English edn. *Gastric Cancer* **1**: 10–24.

7. The Paris endoscopic classification of superficial neoplastic lesions: esophagus, stomach, and colon: November 30 to December 1, 2002. (2003) *Gastrointest Endosc* **58**: S3–S43.

8. Kakeji Y, Yamaguchi S, Yoshida D, *et al.* (2006) Development and assessment of morphologic criteria for diagnosing gastric cancer using confocal endomicroscopy: an *ex vivo* and *in vivo* study. *Endosc* **38**: 886–890.

9. Kitabatake S, Niwa Y, Miyahara R, *et al.* (2006) Confocal endomicroscopy for the diagnosis of gastric cancer *in vivo*. *Endosc* **38**: 1110–1114.

10. Zhang JN, Li YQ, Zhao YA, *et al.* (2008) Classification of gastric pit patterns by confocal endomicroscopy. *Gastrointest Endoscopy* **67**: 843–853.

11. Rugge M, Farinati F, Baffa R, *et al.* (1994) Gastric epithelial dysplasia in the natural history of gastric cancer: a multicenter prospective follow-up study. Interdisciplinary Group on Gastric Epithelial Dysplasia. *Gastroenterology* **107**: 1288–1296.

12. Tsukuma H, Oshima A, Narahara H, Morii T. (2000) Natural history of early gastric cancer: a non-concurrent long term follow-up study. *Gut* **47**: 618–621.

Part 5

SMALL INTESTINE

Chapter 12

Normal Small-Intestinal Mucosa

Histology

The small bowel contains three regions: duodenum, jejunum, and ileum. The normal human small intestine is composed of mucosa, submucosa, muscularis, and serosa. Part of the mucosa and submucosa of the small bowel are thrown into a series of folds by the plicate. This increases the surface area available for absorption.

The mucosa of the small bowel consists of epithelium, lamina propria, and muscularis mucosae. The mucosal surface epithelium and lamina propria of the intestine together project lumina to form villi. Villous morphology includes variations such as finger-like and leaf-like ones. In the duodenum, it is easy to find branched villi. In the distal duodenum and proximal jejunum the villi are longest, while in the mid-small bowel the villi gradually shorten to tubbiness. The epithelium within the basal side of the villi sinks into the lamina propria and forms tubular glands (Fig. 12.1.)

In the mucosa, intestinal villi are covered by simple columnar epithelium and broken into microvilli. The epithelium overlapping villi contain absorptive cells, goblet cells, and endocrine cells. In addition, Paneth cells can be found in tubular glands. Absorptive cells are tall columnar cells with oval, basally located, aligned nuclei, eosinophilic cytoplasm, and a microvillous brush border which can be seen under the light microscope. Goblet cells are scattered among absorptive cells. The bottom of the cells is narrow, while the apical are enlargement which store mucigen droplets, and so the shape resembles a goblet. In HE staining, goblet cells show a large vacuolated. Paneth cells in the basal part of the crypts contain acidophil supranuclear cytoplasmic

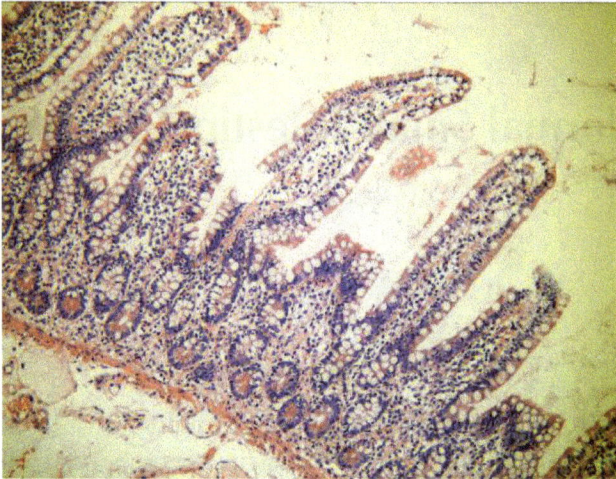

Fig. 12.1.   Longitudinal section of the small bowel (HE × 100). The mucosa of the ileum consists of epithelium, lamina propria, and muscularis mucosae. The mucosal surface epithelium and lamina propria of the intestine together project lumina to form villi whose morphology is finger-like. The epithelium within the basal side of the villi sinks into the lamina propria and forms tubular glands.

granules. Endocrine cells, with a broad base resting on the basement, are triangular in shape (Fig. 12.2.)

The lamina propria usually consists of plasma cells and lymphocytes with a few eosinophils and macrophages. Lymphoid nodules aggregate into Peyer's patches and are uncommon in the duodenum. Each villus has a central connective tissue which contains a central lacteal, capillary network and smooth muscle. Inner circular muscle and outer longitudinal muscle are composed of muscularis mucosae.

Endomicroscopic Imaging of Small Gastrointestinal Mucosa

Because of the restriction of the endoscopic length, we can only use endomicroscopy to observe the descending part of the duodenum and terminal ileum. Intravenous fluorescein is distributed throughout the body, and the mucosal layer of the intestine is able to be observed ranging from the surface to a depth of 250 μm. Beyond that, the

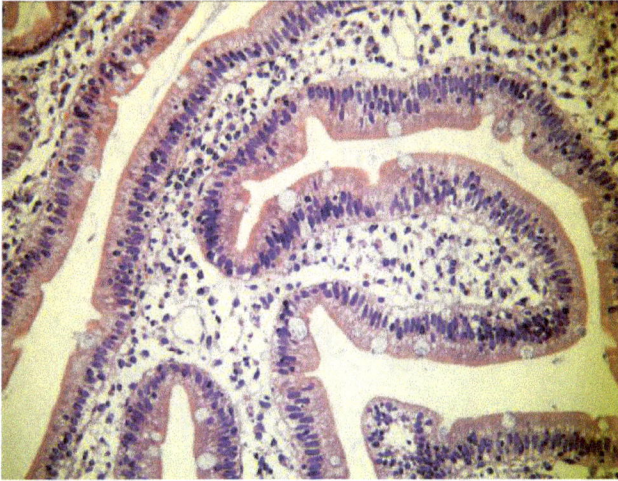

Fig. 12.2. Transverse section of the small bowel (HE × 400). (A) Transverse section of the descendant duodenum, showing that the surface of villi is covered by simple columnar epithelium. The following is lamina propria which contains many capillaries. The epithelium overlapping villi contain absorptive cells and goblet cells. Absorptive cells are tall columnar cells with oval, basally located, aligned nuclei, and a brush border which can be seen on the surface of the cells. Goblet cells, with a shape resembling a goblet, are scattered among absorptive cells.

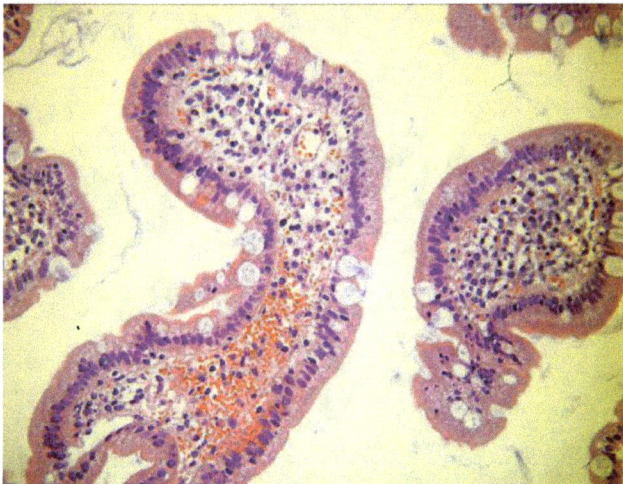

Fig. 12.2(B). Transverse section of the duodenal bulb, identifying absorptive cells with distinguishable brush borders; goblet cells are highly visible.

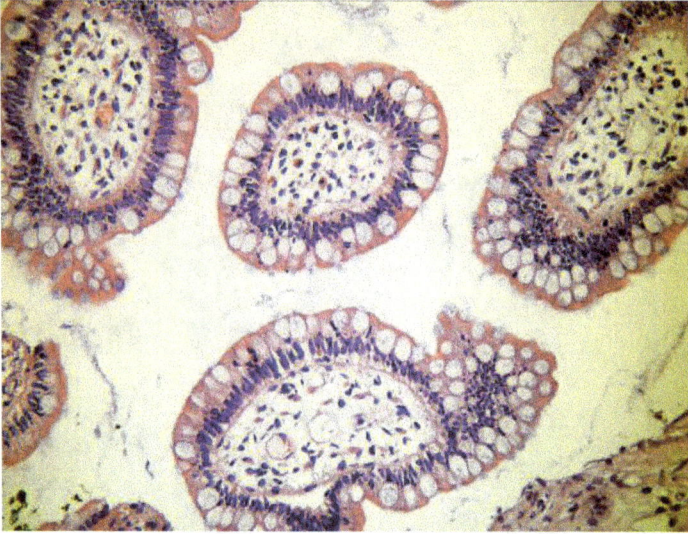

Fig. 12.2(C).   Transverse section of the ileum, showing that goblet cells are increased. Each villus has a central connective tissue which contains a central lacteal capillary network and smooth muscle.

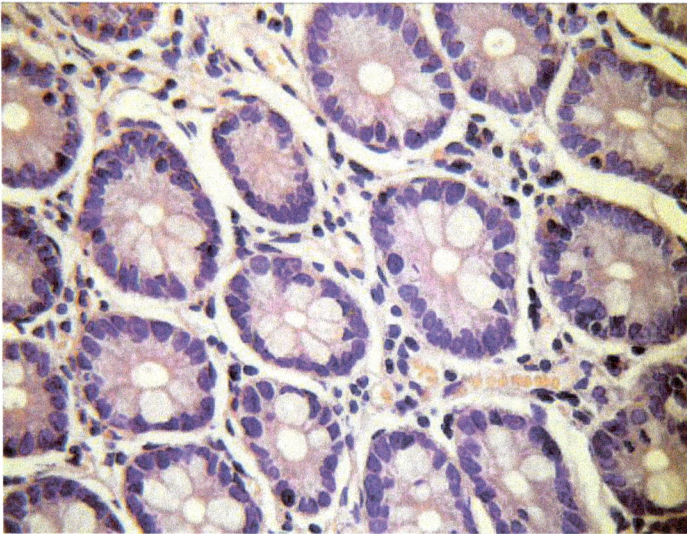

Fig. 12.2(D).   In the lamina propria, tubular glands are composed of absorptive cells, goblet cells, and Paneth cells. Paneth cells in the basal part of the glands contain acidophil supranuclear cytoplasmic granules.

height of the intestinal villi will influence the observation. So, in most cases, only the upper third of the mucosal layer can be revealed. However, some of the deep structure cannot be observed, such as the muscularis and serosa. (Fig. 12.3)

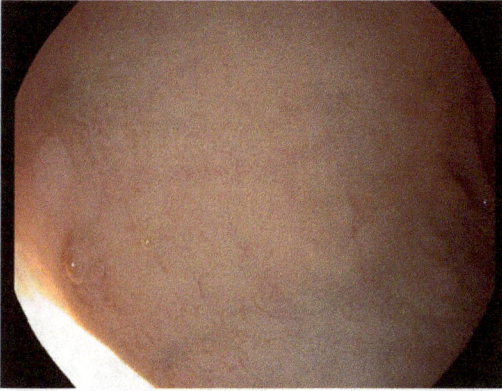

Fig. 12.3. High-definition endoscopy and histology images of the normal duodenal bulb. (A) High-definition endoscopy of the duodenal bulb: the mucosa is smooth and the villi are highly visible.

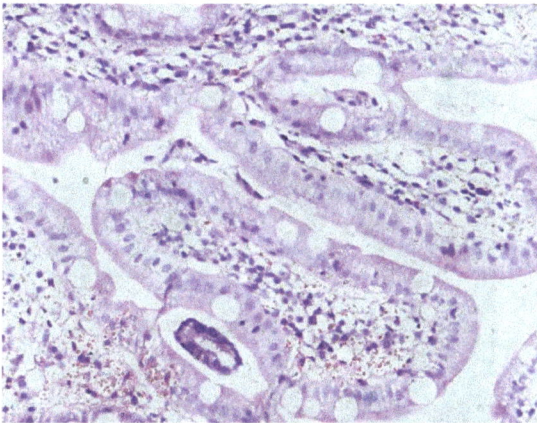

Fig. 12.3(B). Conventional histology of the duodenal bulb architecture, showing absorptive cells, goblet cells, brush border, and lamina propria. Absorptive cells are tall columnar cells with oval, basally located aligned nuclei, and eosinophilic cytoplasm. Goblet cells are scattered among absorptive cells. The bottom of the cells is narrow, while the apical are enlargement which store mucigen droplets, and so the shape resembles a goblet.

After IV administration of fluorescein sodium (a 10% solution), the mucosa of the duodenal and terminal ileum displays finger-like or leaf-like villi that superficially and clearly identify stained goblet cells. (Fig. 12.4)

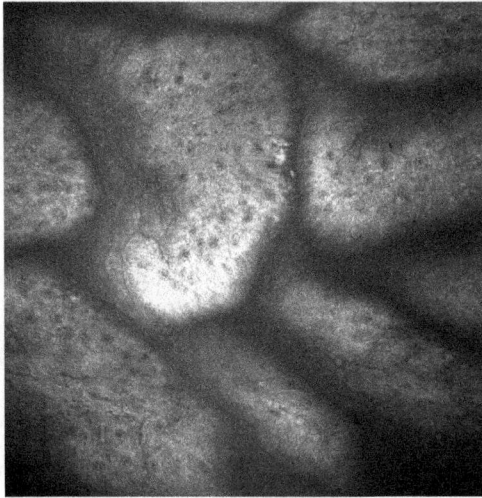

Fig. 12.4.   The surface of the villi. (A) After IV administration of fluorescein sodium (a 10% solution), the mucosa of the duodenal bulb displays finger-like or leaf-like villi that superficially and clearly identify regular-appearing polygonal absorptive cells, and stained goblet cells are scattered among the absorptive cells.

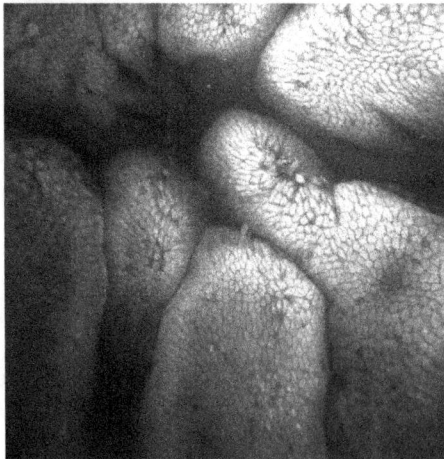

Fig. 12.4(B).   Acriflavine staining enables visualization of the finger-like villi, with regular-appearing absorptive cells and goblet cells.

In the surface mucosal layer, most of the images obtained from CLE reveal a typical villiform shape, with uniform-appearing columnar-lined epithelium and mucus-containing goblet cells. Absorptive cells are tall columnar and slim in shape. The brush border (black line) is present at the outer edge of the bright absorptive cells (Fig. 12.5A)

When acriflavine is used as a contrast medium, it is easy to visualize the nucleus located on the basal side of the absorptive cells (Fig. 12.5B).

In histology goblet cells are displayed very brightly, while in endomicroscopy mucin within cells is shown dark. Goblet cells show a typical target-like appearance, and dark mucin was identified on the apical side of the goblet cells (Fig. 12.6).

In the intermediate layer, endomicroscopy enables the clear and regular-appearing subepithelial capillary network to be visible (Fig. 12.7).

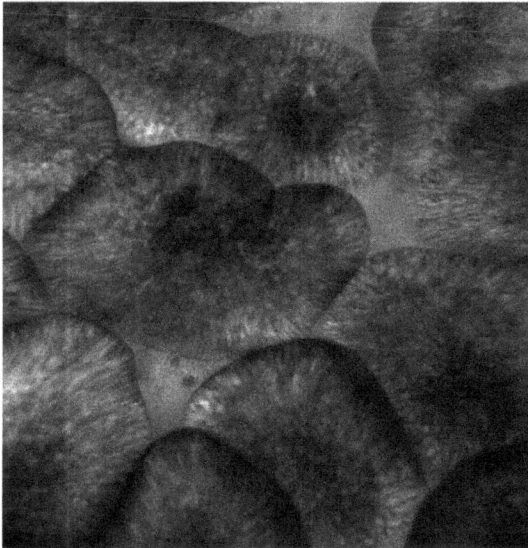

Fig. 12.5. The absorptive cells in the duodenal bulb. (A) When fluorescein sodium (a 10% solution) is used for staining, the absorptive cells show approximately uniform size and shape (tall columnar, slim, and bright), and the black line at the outer edge of the absorptive cells represents the brush border.

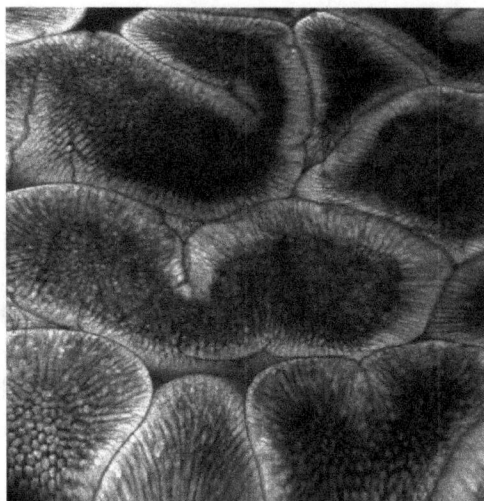

Fig. 12.5(B). The tall columnar and slim absorptive cells and basally located aligned nuclei can be seen with acriflavine-aided endomicroscopy.

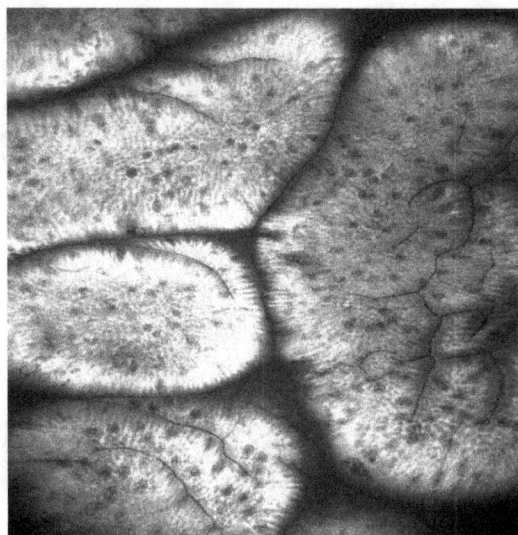

Fig. 12.6. The goblet cells in the duodenal bulb. (A) When fluorescein sodium (10%) is used as a contrast medium, these black and buninoid goblet cells are distributed among the bright absorptive cells, and so that they form a striking contrast.

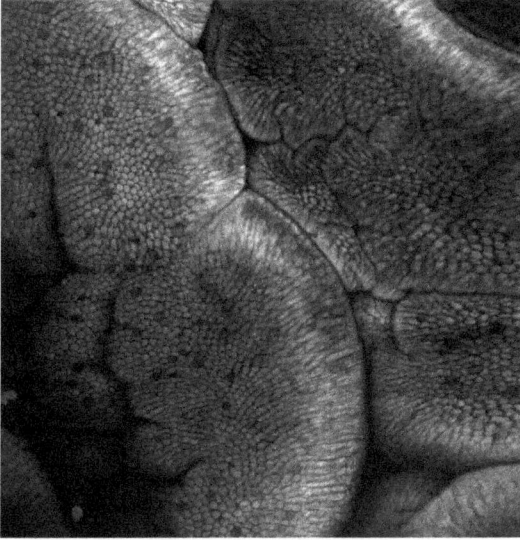

Fig. 12.6(B). However, when acriflavine is used as a contrast medium, goblet cells show a typical targetlike appearance and stain thin.

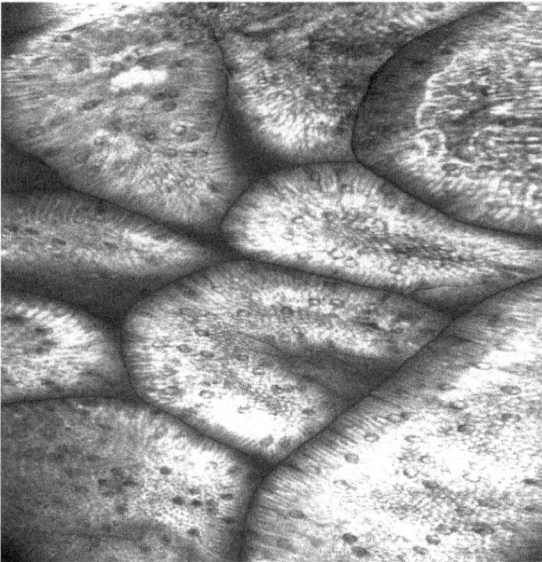

Fig. 12.7. Endomicroscopy especially brings out the capillary architecture within the surface layer and the deep layer of the villi.

Besides, the underlying glands cannot be revealed endomicroscopically among the healthy villi. However, when the villi atrophy (such as from severe inflammation or celiac disease), the glands in the basal part of the villi can be observed.

References

1. Day DW, Jass JR, Price AB, *et al.* (2003) *Morson and Dawson's Gastrointestinal Pathology*, pp. 237–401.
2. Kiesslich R, Galle PR, Neurath MF. (2008) *Atlas of Endomicroscopy.* Springer Medizin Verlag PR.
3. Serra S, Jani PA. (2006) An approach to duodenal biopsies. **59:** 1133–1150.

Chapter 13

Small-Intestinal Inflammation

Malignant neoplasms are rare in the small intestine compared with the colon. This section mainly aims to discuss the inflammatory disorders of the small intestine. The inflammatory disorders are considered to be acquired conditions related to various causes, and different pathological mechanisms may cause the same morphological appearance. Therefore, we can divide them into two main groups: nonspecific inflammation (e.g. duodenitis, pouchitis) and inflammation due to other causes (e.g. celiac disease, Whipple's disease, inflammatory bowel disease).

Nonspecific Duodenitis

Nonspecific duodenitis is mainly secondary to acid injury and *H. pylori* infection. The diagnosis of duodenitis is made when there is infiltration by inflammatory cells with different changes of villous architecture and surface epithelium. Mild duodenitis shows a small increase of chronic inflammatory cells in the lamina propria, associated with slight widening or flattening of villi (Figs. 13.1 and 13.2). Severe duodenitis is characterized by intense inflammatory cell infiltration of the lamina propria and neutrophils into the surface epithelium, together with changes in the villous architecture. Heavy polymorphonuclear invasion is associated with epithelial degeneration, with cytoplasmic vacuolization, intercellular edema, and erosions. These changes are particularly prominent adjacent to a duodenal ulcer (Figs. 13.3 and 13.4).

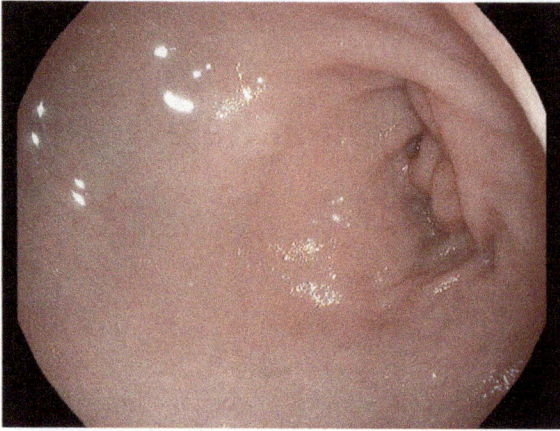

Fig. 13.1.   Endoscopic appearance of mild duodenitis.

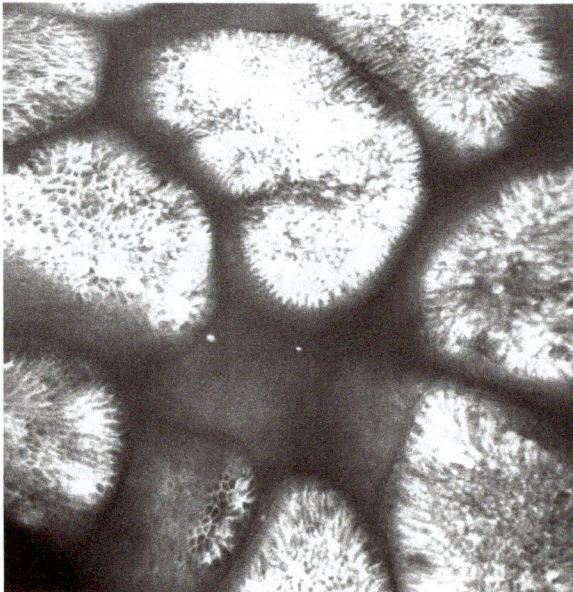

Fig. 13.2.   Mild-to-moderate duodenitis (the surface layer): the villous morphology is still heterogeneous, with fluorescein leakage into spaces among epithelial cells.

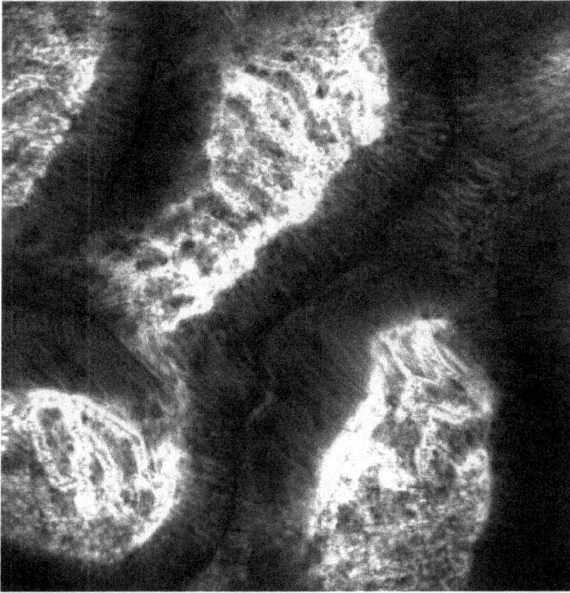

Fig. 13.3. Mild-to-moderate duodenitis (intermediate layer): the presence of mild-to-moderate cellular infiltration in the lamina propria. There is a mild increase in capillary density with tortuosity.

Gastric Metaplasia

Gastric metaplasia of the duodenum is characterized by replacement of intestinal epithelial cells with gastric-type mucous cells. This disorder is largely restricted to the duodenal bulb and distribution is patchy. The foci of gastric epithelial cells contain PAS-positive neutral mucin and lack a brush border. Gastric metaplasia is considered to be an acquired nonspecific response to mucosal injury resulting from gastric acid[1,2] and chronic inflammation.[3,4] It is frequently found at the edge of a duodenal ulcer, and the patches of metaplasia are often colonized by *H. pylori*.[5,6] The diagnosis is based on histological examination of duodenal biopsies and can be highlighted by a combined Alcian blue/periodic acid-Schiff (AB/PAS) stain, where neutral mucin in the gastric epithelium stains red while the combination of acidic and neutral mucins in goblet cells stains blue.

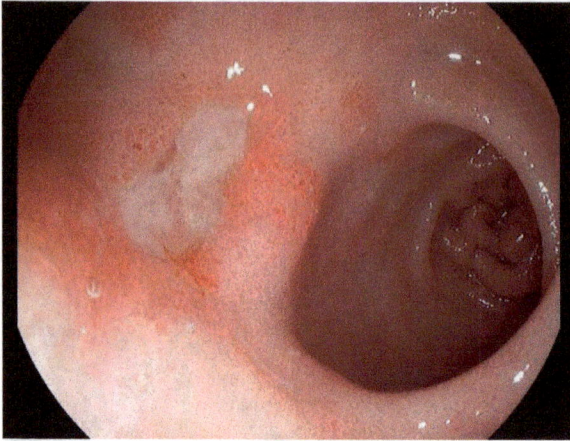

Fig. 13.4.   Endoscopic appearance of severe duodenitis.

The existence and extent of gastric metaplasia can be evaluated accurately *in vivo* by CLE. This is because fluorescein is a pH-dependent dye; different fluorescein signals were shown in different tissues, due to the intracellular pH. The cytoplasm of gastric columnar cells which contain neutral mucin appears darker than normal duodenal columnar cells and can be easily identified (Figs. 13.5–13.6).

Celiac Disease

Celiac disease is considered to be an autoimmune enteropathy triggered by the ingestion of gluten-containing grains.[7]

Pathological changes are mainly found in the duodenal mucosa and in the upper jejunum; serological tests and endoscopic features (a reduction in the number of duodenal folds, scalloping of folds, a mosaic pattern, or nodularity of the mucosa) can help in diagnosis,[8–10] but the sensitivity was not satisfactory. Histological findings on duodenal mucosal samples remain essential for diagnosis.[11] However, because of its patchy nature, the diagnosis can be missed if inadequate biopsies are taken for histological examination. Celiac disease has a wide spectrum of histological abnormalities, ranging from a slight villous flattening to a decreased V:C ratio, crypt hyperplasia, increased

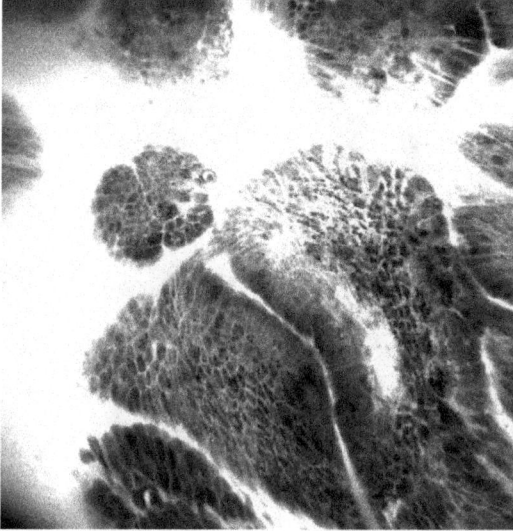

Fig. 13.5. Severe duodenitis (the surface layer): epithelial degeneration, intercellular edema, and gross fluorescein leakage can be observed.

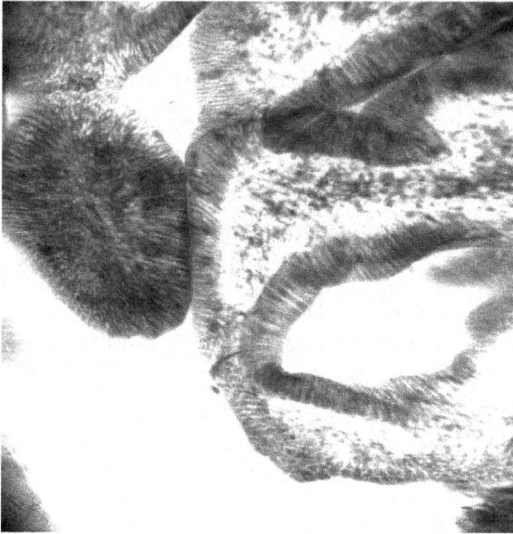

Fig. 13.6. Severe duodenitis (intermediate layer): villi are flattened and irregular in shape, and the crypt opening is present with gross fluorescein extravasation.

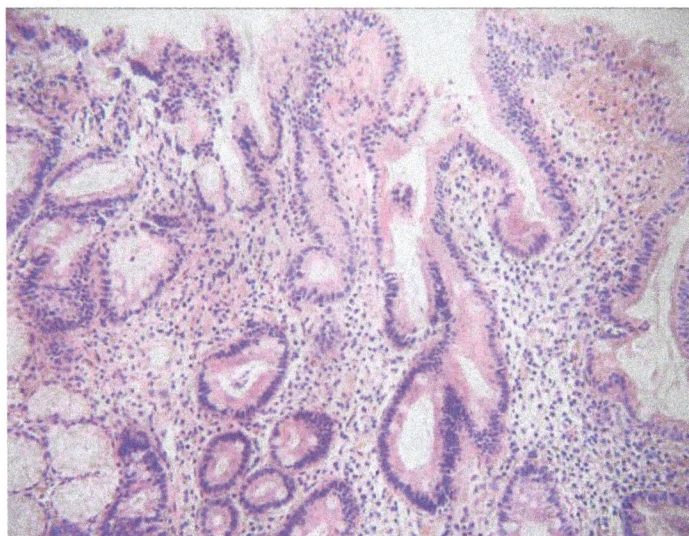

Fig. 13.7. Light micrograph of severe duodenitis with HE staining. The lamina propria shows an increase in the inflammatory cells.

plasma cell and lymphocyte infiltration in the lamina propria, and a marked increase in the IEL count.[12] The current histopathological diagnosis is made using the Marsh criteria as modified by Oberhuber.[13]

CLE allows the visualization of microscopic details of the mucosal surface during endoscopy; it is a potentially useful technique for such patients. The duodenal mucosa can be evaluated by CLE in respect of villous atrophy and crypt hyperplasia (Fig. 13.7). Furthermore, the increased numbers of intraepithelial lymphocytes can be evaluated by topical application of acriflavine.[14,15] However, in those patients without villous atrophy (Marsh I–II), the detection of crypt hyperplasia by CLE is difficult because of the limited imaging depth. Therefore, Marsh II is difficult to diagnose by CLE.

Duodenal Inflammatory Polyps

Duodenal polyp lesions are mainly inflammatory polyps and Brunner's gland hyperplasia. It may be difficult to distinguish them by macroscopic findings. Inflammatory polyps can also be evaluated in the duodenum and terminal ileum by CLE. The villi are usually folded, widened in shape, and hyperplasia of surface columnar epithelium cells can be seen without atypia (Fig. 13.8).

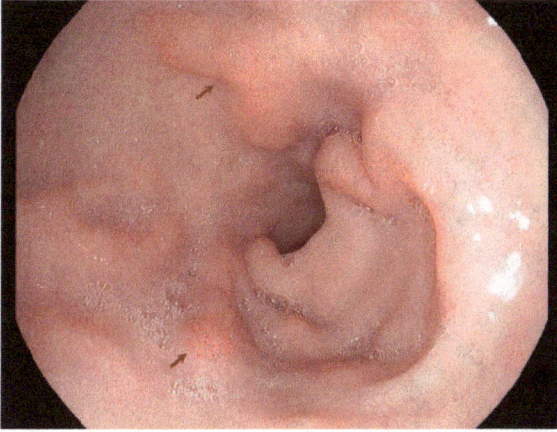

Fig. 13.8.   Endoscopic appearance of visible gastric metaplasia.

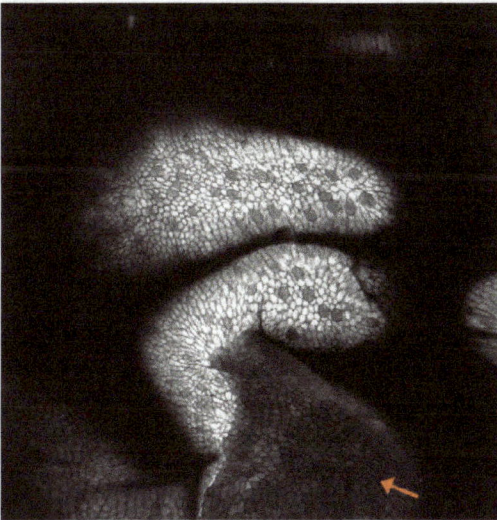

Fig. 13.9.   Focal gastric metaplasia. Enterocytes are replaced by foci of dark gastric-type cells (acriflavine stains).

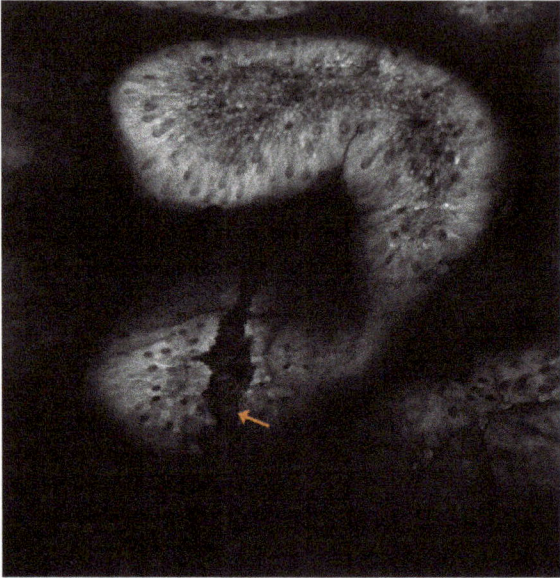

Fig. 13.10. Focal gastric metaplasia. Enterocytes are replaced by foci of dark gastric-type cells (fluorescein stains).

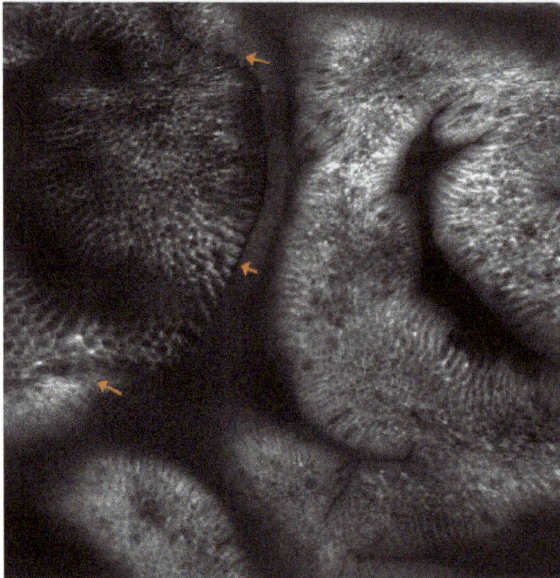

Fig. 13.11. Gastric metaplasia involves several villi, and villi appear blunted. The arrows show the borderline between the metaplasia and the normal area.

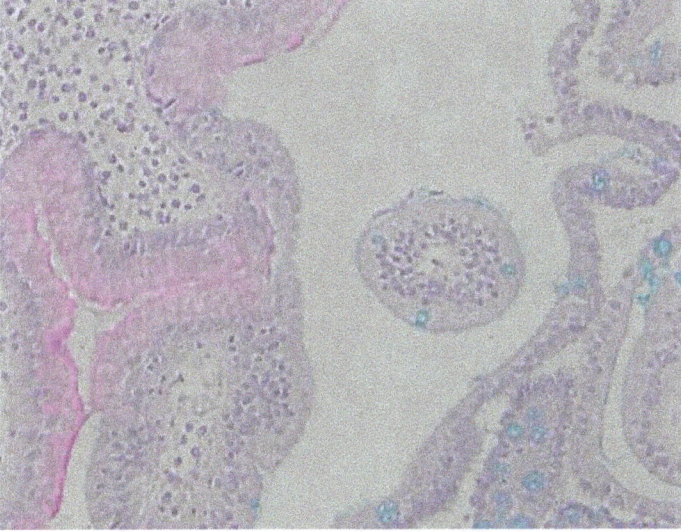

Fig. 13.12. Focal gastric metaplasia. Enterocytes are replaced by foci of gastric-type mucus-secreting cells. Villi are shortened and blunted.

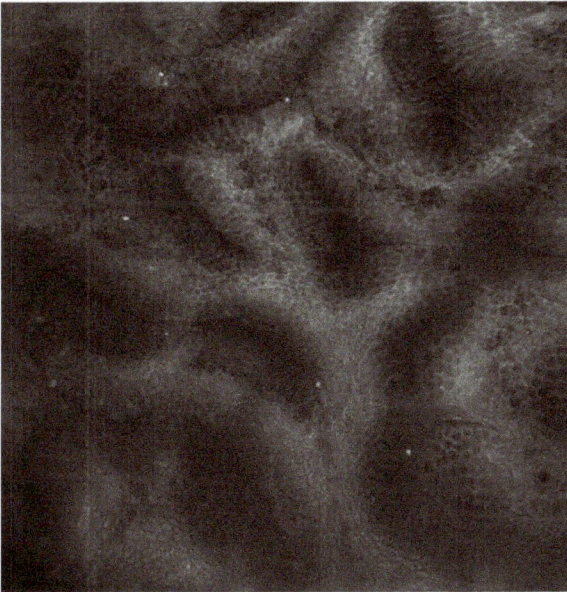

Fig. 13.13. Extensive gastric metaplasia: the musosa is flattened and bulbous in shape. Villi have completely disappeared, instead of the gastric pit.

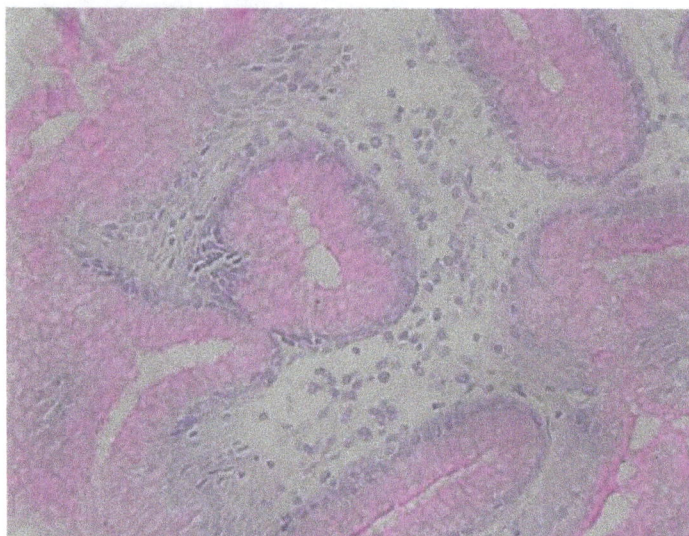

Fig. 13.14.   Corresponding histological specimen of extensive gastric metaplasia.

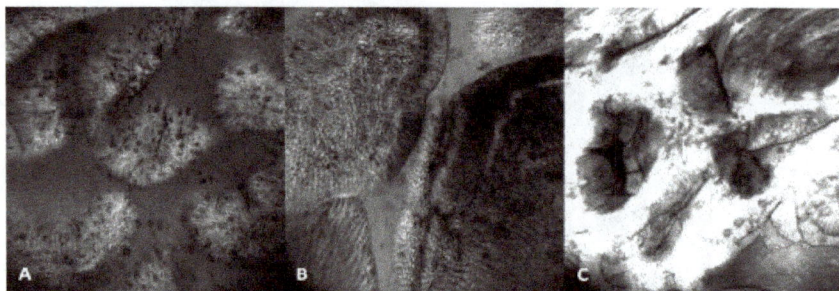

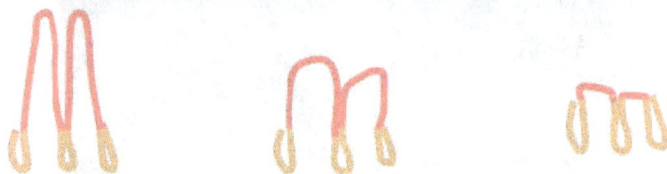

Fig. 13.15.   Celiac disease diagnosed *in vivo* by confocal endomicroscopy. (A) The surface of the villi shows transversal furrows with goblet cells between enterocytes. The villi appear regular, finger-like, and leaf-like. (B) Villous atrophy is defined as a flattening of the surface secondary to the shortening and blunting of villi. The number of villi was decreased. (C) A nearly flat mucosal surface with total villous atrophy and crypt hyperplasia.

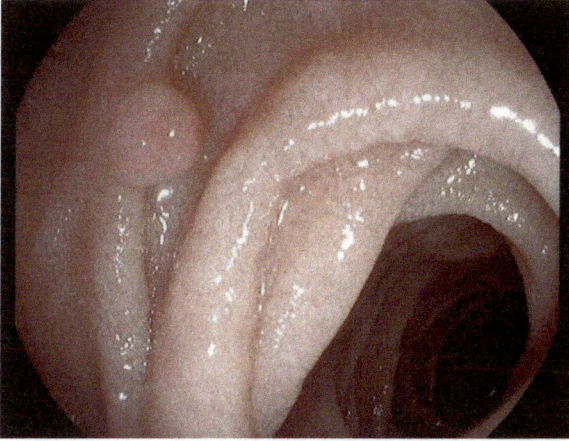

Fig. 13.16. Endoscopic appearance of an inflammatory polyp.

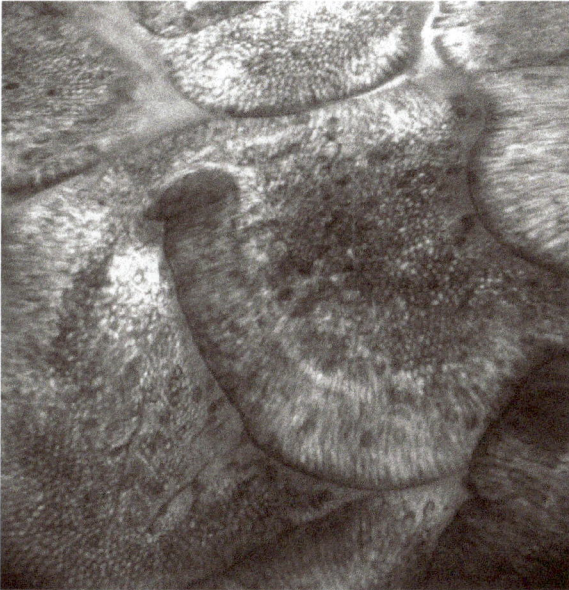

Fig 13.17. Inflammatory polyp. The villi are folded, and there is marked hyperplasia of surface columnar epithelium cells without atypia.

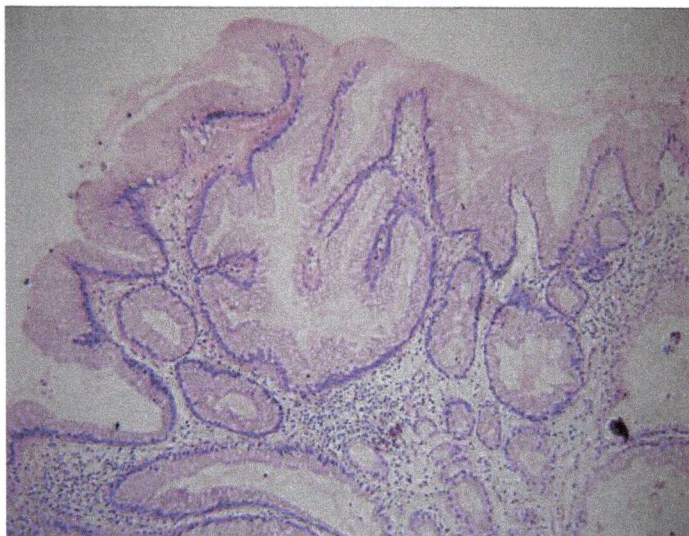

Fig. 13.18. Corresponding histological specimen of an inflammatory polyp.

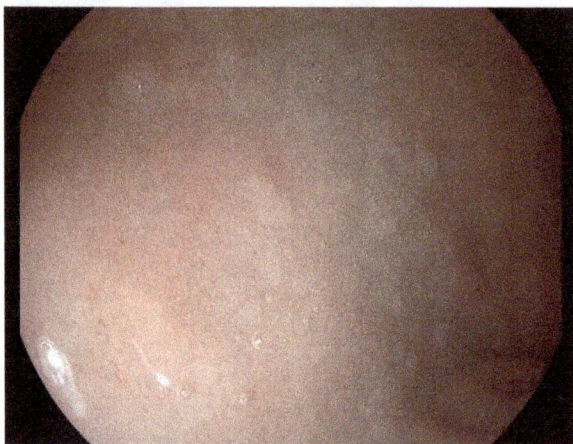

Fig. 13.19. Endoscopic appearance of Brunner's gland hyperplasia.

Brunner's glands are mucin-secreting glands situated in the deep mucosa and submucosa of the duodenum, secreting mucus and pepsinogen in response to acid stimulation. Brunner's gland hyperplasia makes up 10.6% of benign tumors in the duodenum and rarely

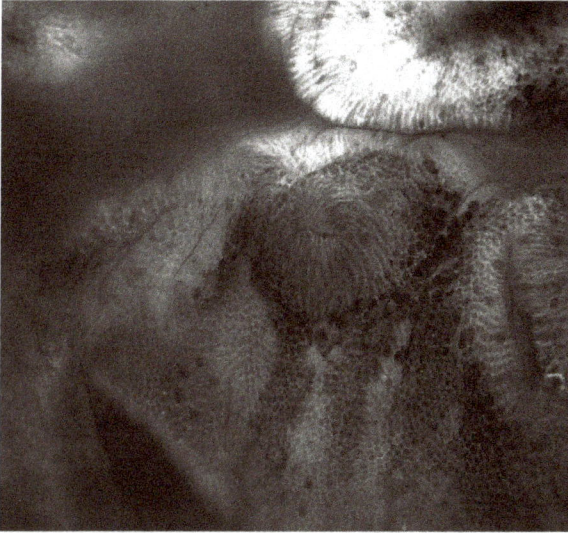

Fig. 13.20. Brunner's gland hyperplasia. A Brunner's gland opening can be observed.

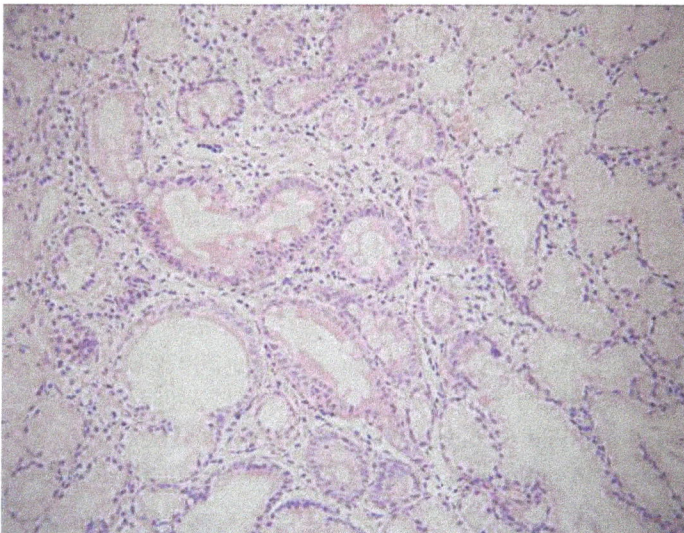

Fig. 13.21. Corresponding histological specimen of Brunner's gland hyperplasia.

presents any symptoms.[16] It is generally polypoid in configuration. Feyrter classified three types of Brunner's gland hyperplasia.[17] Circumscript nodular hyperplasia is the most common type, mainly present in the duodenal bulb, and usually less than 1 cm in size. It is generally found incidentally, because it is small and asymptomatic. A confocal image shows epithelial lesions consisting of clumps of Brunner's glands, and focal cystic changes may be seen.

References

1. Harris A, Gummett P, Walker M, *et al.* (1996) Relation between gastric acid output, *Helicobacter pylori*, and gastric metaplasia in the duodenal bulb. *Gut* **39**: 513–520.

2. Faller G, Dimmler A, Rau T, *et al.* (2004) Evidence for an acid-induced loss of Cdx2 expression in gastric metaplasia in the duodenum. *J Pathol* **203**: 904–908.

3. Voutilainen M, Juhola M, Farkkila M, *et al.* (2003) Gastric metaplasia and chronic inflammation at the duodenal bulb mucosa. *Dig Liver Dis* **35**: 94–98.

4. Urakami Y, Sano T. (2001) Endoscopic duodenitis, gastric metaplasia and *Helicobacter pylori*. *J Gastroenterol Hepatol* **16**: 513–518.

5. Satoh K, Kimura K, Yoshida Y, *et al.* (1993) Relationship between *Helicobacter pylori* colonization and acute inflammation of the duodenal mucosa. *Am J Gastroenterol* **88**: 360–363.

6. Blaser M, Atherton J. (2004) *Helicobacter pylori* persistence: biology and disease. *J Clin Investig* **113**: 321–333.

7. Fasano A, Catassi C. (2001) Current approaches to diagnosis and treatment of celiac disease: an evolving spectrum. *Gastroenterology* **120**: 636–651.

8. Brocchi E, Tomassetti P, Misitano B, *et al.* (2002) Endoscopic markers in adult coeliac disease. *Dig Liver Dis* **34**: 177–182.

9. Jabbari M, Wild G, Goresky CA, *et al.* (1988) Scalloped valvulae conniventes: an endoscopic marker of celiac sprue. *Gastroenterology* **95**: 1518–1522.

10. Brocchi E, Corazza GR, Brusco G, *et al.* (1996) Unsuspected celiac disease diagnosed by endoscopic visualization of duodenal bulb micronodules. *Gastrointest Endosc* **44**: 610–611.

11. Dickey W. (2002) Endoscopy, serology and histology in the diagnosis of coeliac disease. *Dig Liver Dis* **34**: 172–174.

12. Serra S, Jani PA. (2006) An approach to duodenal biopsies: *J Clin Pathol* 1133–1150.

13. Oberhuber G, Granditsch G, Vogelsang H. (1999) The histopathology of coeliac disease: time for a standardized report scheme for pathologists. *Eur J Gastroenterol Hepatol* **11**: 1185–1194.

14. Leong RW, Nguyen NQ, Meredith CG, *et al.* (2008) *In vivo* confocal endomicroscopy in the diagnosis and evaluation of celiac disease. *Gastroenterology* **135**: 1870–1876.

15. Günther U, Daum S, Heller F, *et al.* (2010) Diagnostic value of confocal endomicroscopy in celiac disease. *Endoscopy* **42**: 197–202.

16. Peetz ME, Moseley HS. (1989) Brunner's gland hyperplasia. *Am Surg.* **55**: 474–477.

17. Feyrter F. (1938) Uber wucherunger der Brunnerschen Drusen. *Virchows Arch* **293**: 509–526.

Part 6

COLON

Chapter 14

Normal Colonic Mucosa

Histology

The surface of colon mucosa consists of thousands of crypts of uniform size and shape. The crypts are covered mainly by two types of cells: absorptive cells and goblet cells. Epithelial cells originate from the base of the crypts and migrate to the openings, and are shed in the middle of neighboring crypts, forming grooves defining the boundaries of all the crypts. The openings of the crypts are distributed evenly on the surface of the mucosa. The base of each crypt extends down in the muscularis mucosa. The spaces between the crypts are filled with lamina propria containing microvessels, nerves, smooth muscle, lymphocytes, and so on. In normal conditions, the shape and distribution of the crypts are regular and uniform. Microvessels surrounding the crypts form a honeycomb-like network within the lamina propria[1] (Fig. 14.1).

Endomicroscopic Imaging of Normal Colonic Mucosa

The *en face* endomicroscopic image of colon mucosa shows regularly arranged round crypts. The openings of the crypts are black holes at the center of the crypts. Goblet cells can be easily identified by either fluorescein or acriflavine[2] (Figs. 14.2 and 14.3). They are more abundant in the superficial layers than in the deeper layers. Fluorescein-stained microvessels surrounding the crypts form a honeycomb-like network. Basement membrane separating epithelium from lamina propria can be identified more easily in deeper layers of CLE images[3] (Fig. 14.4). Grooves which are hard to see in histological slices are visible in CLE images acquired from distal colon mucosa (Fig. 14.5).

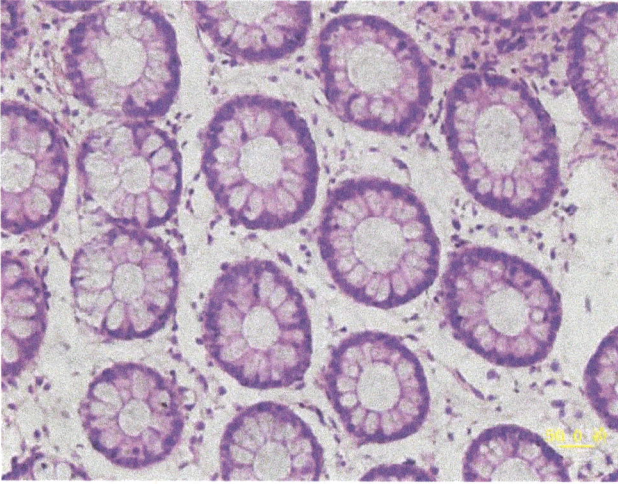

Fig. 14.1. Histology of normal colonic musoca. The colonic mucosa contains round crypts of uniform size. Each crypt is covered by absorptive cells and goblet cells. Lamina propria in the spaces among the crypts contains lymphocytes.

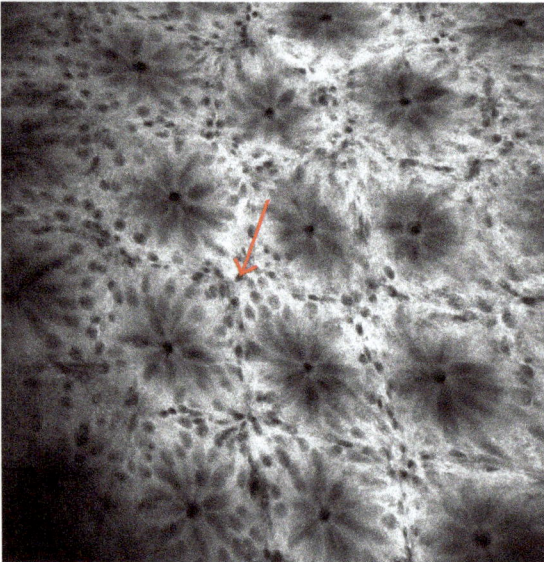

Fig. 14.2. CLE image showing the superficial layer of rectal mucosa (10% fluorescein sodium alone). Grooves defining the boundaries of the crypts are highly visible (*arrow*).

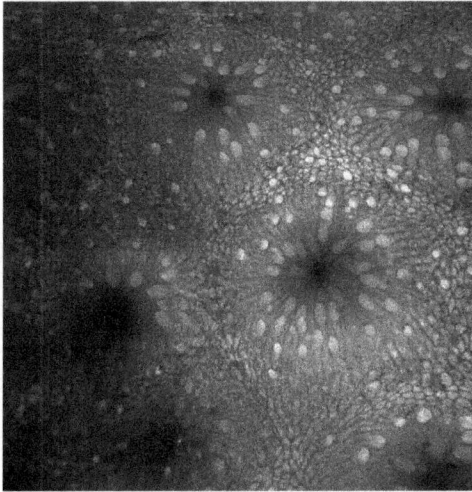

Fig. 14.3. CLE image showing the superficial layer of colonic mucosa (10% fluorescein sodium and 0.02% acriflavine together). The openings of the crypts are shown as black holes. Goblet cells are larger and brighter than the surrounding absorptive cells.

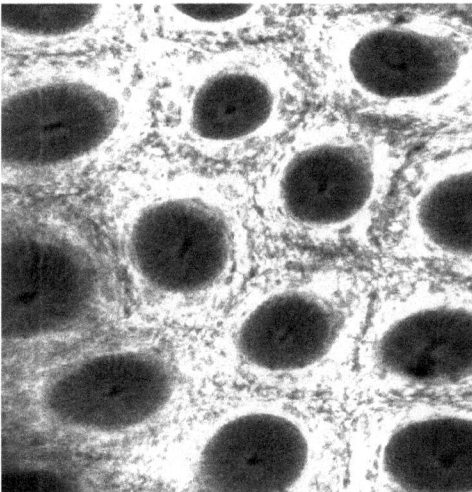

Fig. 14.4. CLE image showing the deeper layer of colonic mucosa (10% fluorescein sodium alone). The number of goblet cells decreases. Microvessels surrounding the crypts form a honeycomb-like network in the lamina propria.

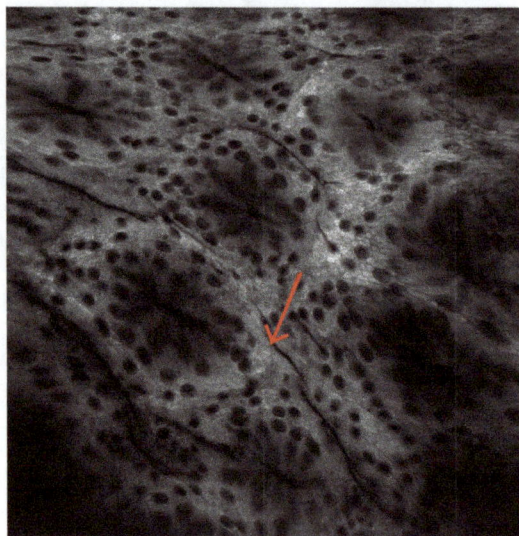

Fig. 14.5. CLE image showing the superficial layer of colonic mucosa (10% fluorescein sodium alone). Colonic crypts are round and regularly arranged. Goblet cells are shown as darker dots compared to the surrounding epithelium (*arrow*).

References

1. Day DW, Jass JR, Price AB, *et al.* (2003) *Morson and Dawson's Gastrointestinal Pathology*, pp. 437–439.
2. Kiesslich R, Goetz M, Angus EM, *et al.* (2007) Identification of epithelial gaps in human small and large intestine by confocal endomicroscopy. *Gastroenterology* **133**: 1769–1778.
3. Kiesslich R, Galle PR, Neurath MF. (2008) *Atlas of Endomicroscopy*, pp. 49–51.

Chapter 15

Ulcerative Colitis

The endoscopic assessment of patients with ulcerative colitis (UC) is essential in the diagnosis, treatment decision, and prediction of prognosis. Currently the application of endomicroscopy in UC remains in two main areas: inflammation activity assessment and identification of colitis associated intraepithelial neoplasia (IN).

Inflammation Activity Assessment

The primary object of endoscopic assessment of patients with UC is to differentiate active from silent, as patients with active inflammation are more likely to relapse than those whose conditions are silent. And patients with long-standing active inflammation are at higher risk of colorectal neoplasia.[1,2]

Mucosa with apparent changes such as erosion and ulcer is easy to determine as active inflammation. However, a considerable proportion of active inflammation could not be identified by conventional white-light endoscopy. Advanced endoscopy techniques such as chromoscopy and high-magnification endoscopy could increase the accuracy of diagnosis of inflammation activity. However, histological evidence of neutrophil infiltration in epithelium remains the gold standard for active inflammation. Combination of advanced endoscopy and endomicroscopy is an ideal procedure for predicting the histology, in which advanced endoscopy reveals the minimal mucosal changes as targets and endomicroscopy determines their *in vivo* histology.

The Mainz criteria classify the inflammation activity into three degrees — none, mild-to-moderate, and severe — according to three categories, which are crypt architecture, cellular infiltration, and vessel architecture (Table 15.1). Kiesslich *et al.* reported that the overall agreement between CLE prediction of disease activity and histological findings was 92.5%, while white-light endoscopy achieved only an agreement of 58.9%.[3]

Watanabe *et al.* described that the crypts of normal colorectal mucosa were small, round, and regularly arranged, and the crypt lumens of the colorectal glands were small and round. The crypts of colorectal mucosa in nonactive UC were small, round, and slightly irregular in arrangement, and the crypt lumens of the colorectal glands were small and round. Inflammatory cells and capillaries were visible in the lamina propria. The crypts of colorectal mucosa in active UC were large, variously shaped, and irregular in arrangement.[4]

The authors proposed a simplified, four-grade classification for assessing the inflammation activity in UC by CLE. Type A and type B are considered as normal and chronic inflammation respectively, and type C and type D as active inflammation (Figs. 15.1–15.8). Descriptions of the four types are shown in Table 15.2. The results showed that CLE is superior to conventional colonoscopy in assessment

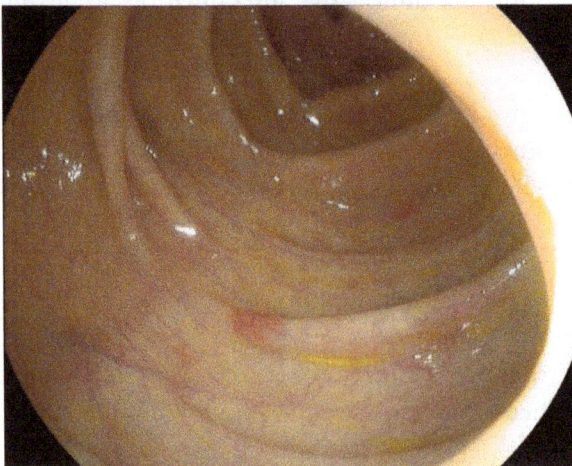

Fig. 15.1. High definition colonoscopy image of UC at the silent stage: smooth mucosa with visible vessels and small areas of erythema.

Table 15.1. Mainz's Classification for Predicting the Activity of Inflammation in UC[3]

Grading of Inflammation	Crypt Architecture	Cellular Infiltration	Vessel Architecture
No	Regular luminal openings and distributi on of crypts covered by a homogeneous layer of epithelial cells, including goblet cells.	Absent	Normal honeycomb-like appearance that displays a network of capillaries outlining the stroma surrounding the luminal openings of the crypts.
Mild-to-moderate	Differences in shape, size, and distribution of crypts; increased distances between crypts, focal crypt destruction.	Present: < 50% of crypts involved.	Mild-to-moderate increase in capillaries; dilated and distorted capillaries.
Severe	Unequivocal crypt destruction.	Present: >50% of crypts involved.	Marked increase in dilated and distorted capillaries; leakage of fluorescein.

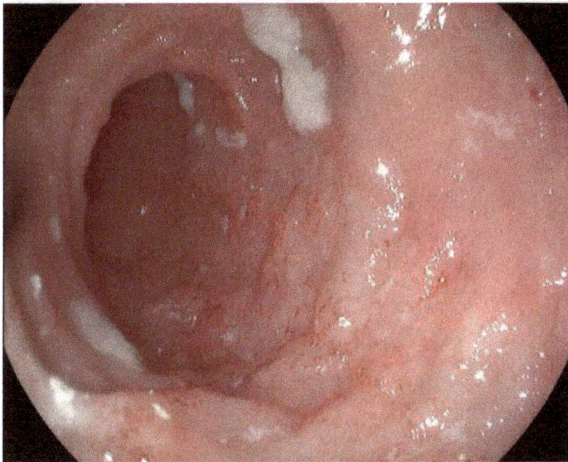

Fig. 15.2.   High-definition colonoscopy image of UC at the active stage: inflamed mucosa with obvious ulcer and erosion.

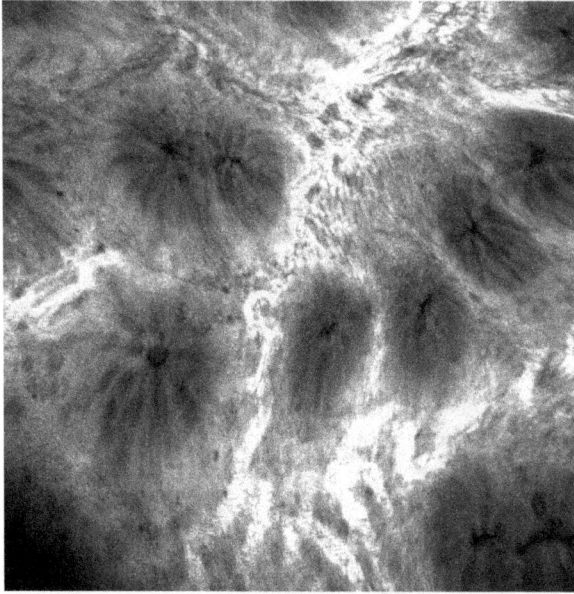

Fig. 15.3. CLE image of UC at the silent stage. The only crypt architecture alteration is irregular arrangement of crypts. The size and shape of the crypts are generally normal.

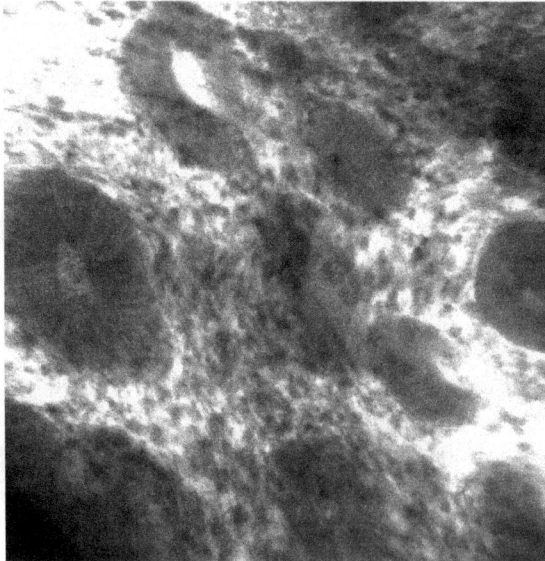

Fig. 15.4. CLE images of UC at the active stage. Figure shows the destruction of crypts and cell infiltration.

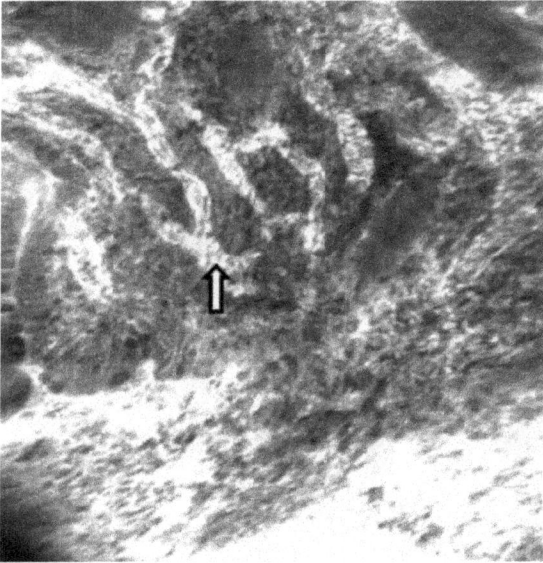

Fig. 15.5.   CLE images of UC at the active stage. Figure shows the vessel with increased number and diameter and fluorescein leakage.

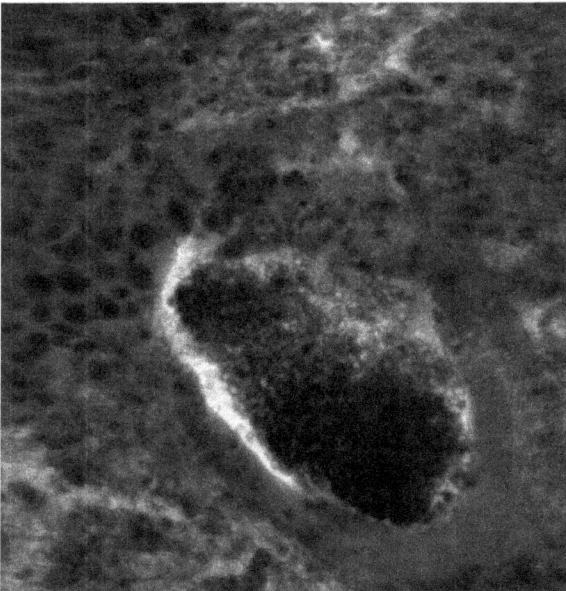

Fig. 15.6.   CLE images of UC at the active stage. Figure shows a single significantly dilated crypt filled with abscess.

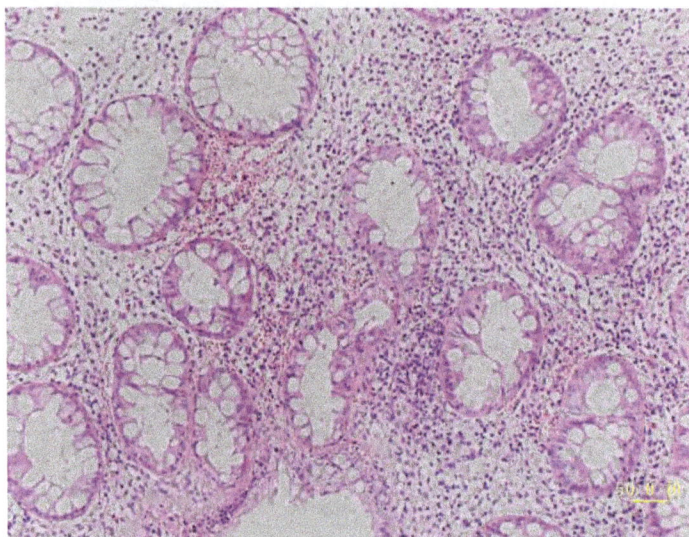

Fig. 15.7. Histological image of UC at the silent stage, showing an irregular arrangement of crypts with sporadic crypt fusions. The crypts are generally normal in size and shape.

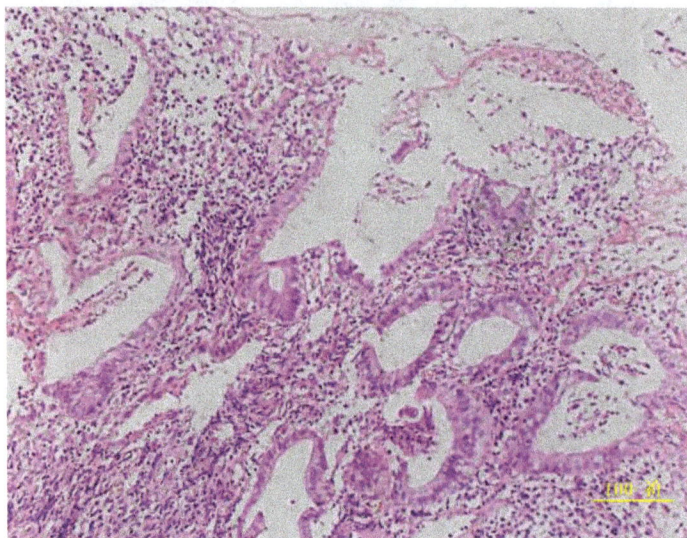

Fig. 15.8. Histological image of UC at the active stage showing the crypt destruction and crypt abscess.

Table 15.2.   Qilu's Classification of Crypt Architecture by CLE Assessment in UC[5]

CLE Crypt Architecture	Description
A	Regular arrangement and size of crypts.
B	Irregular arrangement of crypts; enlarged spaces between crypts.
C	Dilation of crypt openings, more irregular arrangement of crypts, and enlarged spaces between crypts other than type B.
D	Crypt destruction and/or crypt abscess.

of inflammation activity, especially for patients whose conditions appear to be silent under conventional white-light colonoscopy.[5]

Identification of Colitis-associated IN

Patients with a long history of UC have higher risks of colorectal cancer. It was reported that the prevalence of UC-related colorectal cancer was 7% in 20 years and 12% in 30 years. Evidence-based practice suggests that patients with a history of UC longer than 8 years should undergo whole colonoscopy every 1–2 years.[6] Identification and treatment of early stage colorectal cancer or precancerous lesions such as IN could improve the prognosis of UC-related colorectal cancer.

Application of CLE in surveillance of IN is usually combined with other red-flag techniques, such as chromoscopy, because currently CLE itself has no advantage of finding small lesions over conventional colonoscopy. The role of CLE is to confirm whether the lesions found under chromoscopy are INs in a manner of *in vivo* histology diagnosis. Kiesslich *et al.* reported that chromoscopy-guided CLE increased the diagnostic yield of IN in UC by 4.75 times over chromoscopy alone, and a smaller number of biopsies were needed. According to the Mainz criteria, CLE features of IN are a ridge-lined irregular epithelial layer with loss of crypts and goblet cells, irregular cell architecture with little or no mucin, dilated and distorted vessels with increased leakage, and irregular architecture with little or no orientation to adjunct tissues (Table 15.3) (Figs. 15.9–15.11).

Table 15.3. Confocal Pattern Classification for Predicting Colorectal Pathology in Circumscribed Lesions on Chromoscopy[3]

Grading	Crypt Architecture	Vessel Architecture
Normal	Regular luminal openings and distribution of the crypts convered by a homogeneous layer of epithelial cells, including goblet cells.	Honeycomb-like appearance that displays a network of capillaries outlining the stroma surrounding the luminal openings of the crypts.
Regeneration	Star-shaped luminal crypt openings or focal aggregation of regular-shaped crypts with a regular reduced amount of goblet cells.	Honeycomb-like appearance with no or mild increase in the number of capillaries.
Neoplasia	Ridge-lined irregular epithelial layer with loss of crypts and goblet cells, irregular cell architecture with little or no mucin.	Dilated and distorted vessels with increased leakage, irregular architecture with little or no orientation to adjunct tissue.

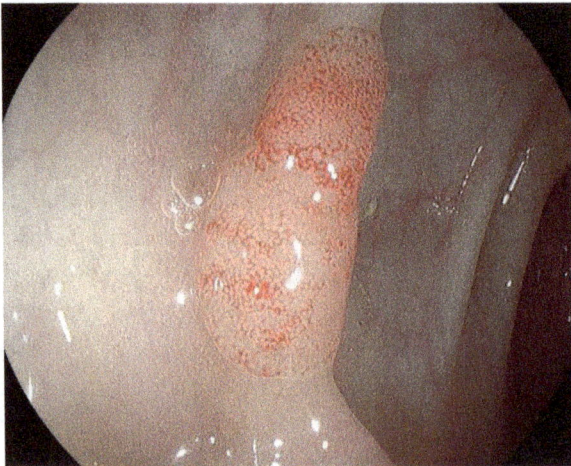

Figure 15.9. High definition colonoscopy image of a flat lesion found in a patient with a long history of UC. The enlarged and irregularly arranged crypts along with an increased blood supply are evident.

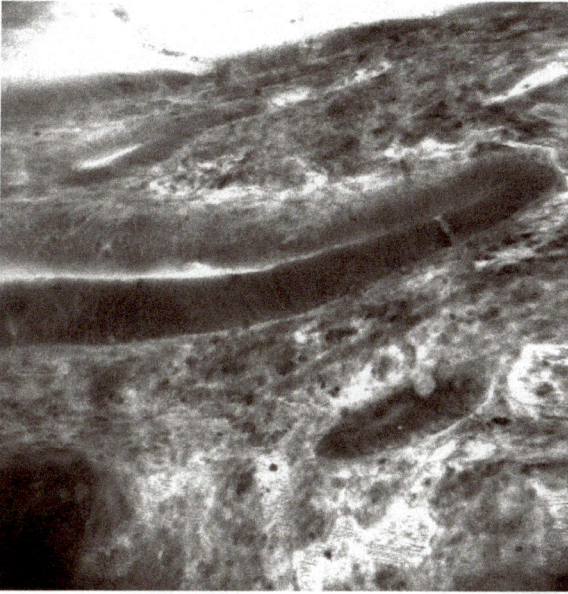

Fig. 15.10. CLE image of the lesion, showing ridge-like epithelium with loss of crypts and goblet cells, irregular cell architecture with little or no mucin, and dilated and distorted vessels.

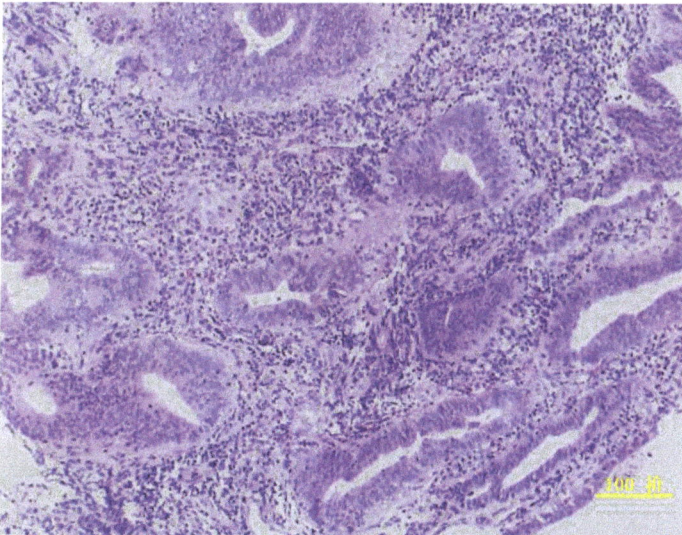

Fig. 15.11. Corresponding histological image of the lesion showing loss of crypts and goblet cells and ridge-like epithelial cell lines.

References

1. Rutter M, Saunders B, Wilkinson K, *et al* (2004). Severity of inflammation is a risk factor for colorectal neoplasia in ulcerative colitis. *Gastroenterology* **126**: 451–459.

2. Gupta RB, Harpaz N, Itzkowitz S, *et al* (2007). Histologic inflammation is a risk factor for progression to colorectal neoplasia in ulcerative colitis: a cohort study. *Gastroenterology* **133**: 1099–1105; quiz 1340–1341.

3. Kiesslich R, Goetz M, Lammersdorf K, *et al.* (2007) Chromoscopy-guided endomicroscopy increases the diagnostic yield of intraepithelial neoplasia in ulcerative colitis. *Gastroenterology* **132**: 874–882.

4. Watanabe O, Ando T, Maeda O, *et al.* (2008) Confocal endomicroscopy in patients with ulcerative colitis. *J Gastroenterol Hepatol* **23**(Suppl 2): S286-S290.

5. Li CQ, Xie XJ, Yu T, *et al.* (2009) Classification of inflammation activity in ulcerative colitis by confocal laser endomicroscopy. *Am J Gastroenterol.*

6. McDonald J, Feagan B, Burroughs A (2004). *Evidence-Based Gastroenterology and Hepatology*, 2nd ed.

Chapter 16

Colorectal Polyps

To improve the prognosis of colorectal cancer, surveillance and treatment of early-stage colorectal cancer and precancerous lesions such as adenomas are cost-effective.[1] According to the adenoma–carcinoma sequence, the identification and removal of colorectal adenomas is effective in reducing the morbidity and mortality of colorectal cancer.[2] Because the most common macroscopic type of colorectal adenoma appears to be the polyp, the removal of all colorectal polyps found during colonoscopy is recommended. However, given that a considerable proportion of colorectal polyps are hyperplastic, with little or no potential for malignancy, the removal of all polyps could increase the risk of unnecessary complications and health care costs.

Advanced White-Light Endoscopy

Real-time colonoscopy evaluation predicting histological diagnosis can assist in the "on-table" diagnosis. In recent years, high-resolution endoscopy or chromoendoscopy has been used in the differential diagnosis of adenomas and hyperplastic polyps. Real-time endoscopy diagnosis of colorectal adenomas appears promising. Most studies used the Kudo classification of five pit patterns in colorectal mucosa, with type II associated with hyperplasia and pit patterns > III associated with neoplasia.[3] The Kudo classification of colorectal lesions is shown in Table 16.1. Examples of high-definition endoscopy images showing hyperplasia and neoplasia are Figs. 16.1 and 16.2.

Table 16.1.   Kudo Classification of Colorectal Lesions

Pit Pattern Type	Characteristics
I	Roundish pits
II	Stellar or papillary pits
III S	Small roundish or tubular pits (smaller than type I pits)
III L	Large roundish or tubular pits (larger than type I pits)
IV	Branch-like or gyrus-like pits
V	Nonstructured pits

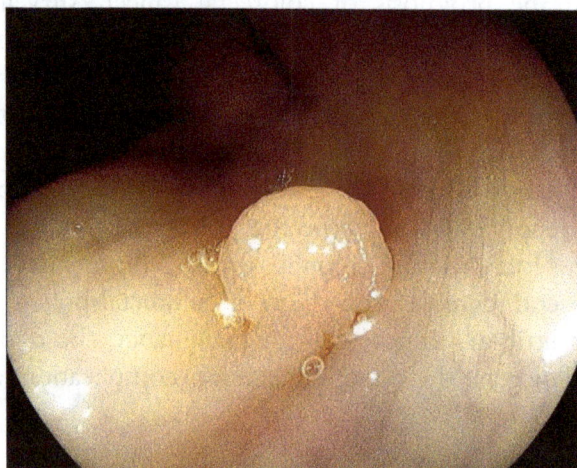

Fig. 16.1.   High-definition endoscopy image of a hyperplastic polyp with Kudo type II.

Confocal Laser Endomicroscopy

There are two major studies on real-time CLE diagnosis of colorectal polyps, with promising results. One of them applied Mainz's criteria using probe-based CLE (pCLE),[4] and the other applied systematic criteria mirroring histology using integrated CLE.[5]

Mainz's criteria

Details of Mainz's criteria for diagnosing colorectal neoplasia can be seen in the previous section. The criteria were first developed for the diagnosis

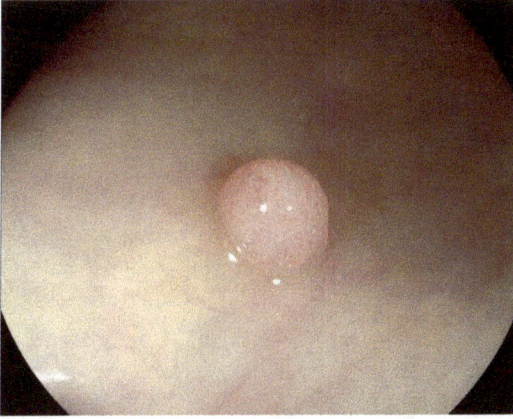

Fig. 16.2. High-definition endoscopy image of an adenoma with Kudo type II.

of neoplasia in patients with ulcerative colitis. Buchner *et al.*[4] applied them to the diagnosis of colorectal polyps to differentiate the neoplastic polyps from the nonneoplastic ones using pCLE. The study included 119 colorectal lesions in 75 patients. The sensitivity and specificity of pCLE were 91% and 76%, respectively. The authors also compared pCLE with two modes of virtual chromoscopy: NBI (narrow band imaging) and FICE (Fuji Intelligent Chromo Endoscopy), with no significant difference in the diagnostic yields between pCLE and virtual chromoscopy.

Sanduleanu's criteria

Sanduleanu *et al.* developed not only a systematic classification of colorectal lesions by using CLE, but also an adenoma dysplasia score (ADS) system to discriminate high-grade dysplasia (HGD) from low-grade dysplasia (LGD). Unlike Mainz's criteria, the colorectal lesions are classified into normal mucosa, nonadenomatous polyps, and adenomatous polyps, and cytonuclear features are important in the differentiation of colorectal polyps. For the 116 lesions from 72 patients included in their study, IN and cancer could be predicted *in vivo* with a sensitivity of 97.3%, and a specificity of 92.8%; ADS ≥ 5 discriminated HGD from LGD with 93.7% sensitivity, 97.7% specificity, and 96.7% accuracy. Details of the criteria and the ADS system are shown in Tables 16.2 and 16.3, respectively.

Table 16.2.   Systematic Classification of Colorectal Lesions by Using CLE

	General Architecture	Cytonuclear Features
Normal mucosa	• Regular (uniform) architecture of surface and glandular epithelium. • Regular honeycomb-like appearance of the vascular pattern.	• Epithelial cells are uniformly lined up along the basement membrane. • Normal cell polarity of surface and glandular epithelium; normal aspect of mucin-producing goblet cells (epithelial cell maturation).
Nonadenomatous polyps	• Slightly disturbed architecture: enlarged, branch-like, elongated crypts (HP, IP). • Increased number of cells in the crypts (mucosal folding, "stellar" aspect) (HP). • Mild alterations of the vascular pattern: faint aspect (HP) or slightly dilated, irregular vessels (IP). • Inflammatory infiltrate of lamina propria; decreased crypt/stroma ratio (IP).	• Epithelial cells are morphologically normal; preserved cell polarity. • Depletion of goblet cells.
Adenomatous polyps	• Disturbed architecture: mild irregularity of the crypts (LGD, SA), eventual villous transformation, simple-to-complex crowding (HGD), causing an increased crypt/stroma ratio to completely altered morphology; crypt destruction (IC). • Mild-to-moderate alterations of the vascular pattern; dilated vessels, irregular aspect (LGD, HGD); neoangiogenesis, with capillary leakage (IC).	• Incomplete to lack of epithelial surface maturation (LGD, HGD, IC). • Slight cytonuclear atypia; basally localized, "pencillate" nuclei, loss of cell polarity with pseudostratification (LGD, SA) to severe cytonuclear atypia; more apically localized, enlarged, roundish nuclei, depletion of goblet cells (HGD). • Islands of malignant cells (IC).

Table 16.3. ADS System for Discriminating HGD from LGD During Endomicroscopy Examination

	LGD	HGD
Epithelial surface maturation	0–1	1–2
0. Normal		
1. Incomplete maturation		
2. Lack of epithelial surface maturation		
Crypt architecture	0–1	1–2
0. Normal		
1. Enlarged, slightly crowded crypts		
2. Crowding, distorted crypts		
Vascular pattern	0–1	1–2
0. Normal		
1. Slightly increased vascular pattern, preserved hexagonal pattern		
2. Increased, distorted vessels		
Cytonuclear atypia	1	2
0. Basal, regular nuclei		
1. Pseudostratification of irregular, pencillate nuclei		
2. Pseudostratification of irregular, large, round, more apically localized nuclei		
Adenoma dysplasia score	1–4	5–8

Newly simplified criteria

Both Mainz's and Sanduleanu's criteria are systematic and composed of categories mirroring histology. For Sanduleanu's criteria, double-staining with fluorescein and acriflavine together is needed for the cytonuclear evaluation. Although not studied in humans, acriflavine was shown to carry a risk for mutagenicity in experimental data. What about simplified criteria with fluorescein alone? We developed simplified criteria based on evaluation of CLE images of 35 polyps with known histology and reviews of published criteria. The simplified criteria have only three categories, such as goblet cell depletion, villous architecture, and microvascular alterations (Table 16.4). A polyp with any of the three features under CLE would be diagnosed as adenoma. The sensitivity and specificity of the simplified criteria in diagnosis of adenoma were 93.9% and 95.9%, respectively. Examples of hyperplastic polyps and adenoma are shown in Figs. 16.3–16.6 (CLE) and Figs. 16.7–16.9 (histology).

Table 16.4. Simplified Criteria for Diagnosis of Colorectal Adenoma

Category	Characteristics
Goblet cell depletion	Homogeneous darker epithelium of colonic crypts
Villous architecture	Replacement of normal crypts by villus-like architecture in the colon
Microvascular alterations	Increased density and caliber of the microvessels with irregular fluorescein leakage in the lamina propria

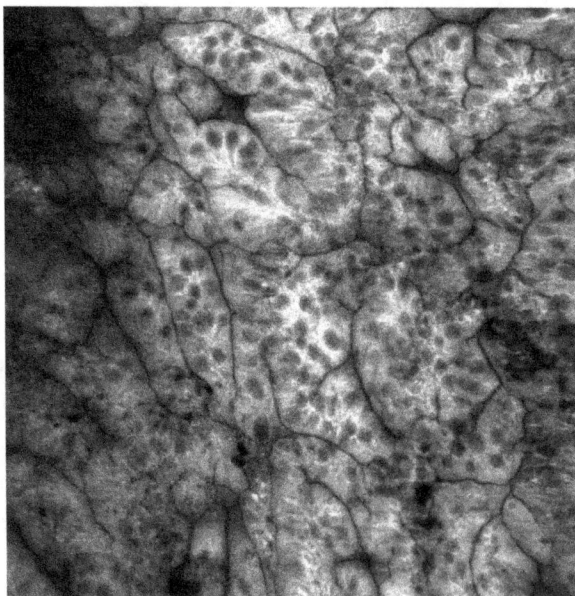

Fig. 16.3. CLE image of a hyperplastic polyp. The crypts with star-shaped openings are covered by both abundant absorptive cells and goblet cells.

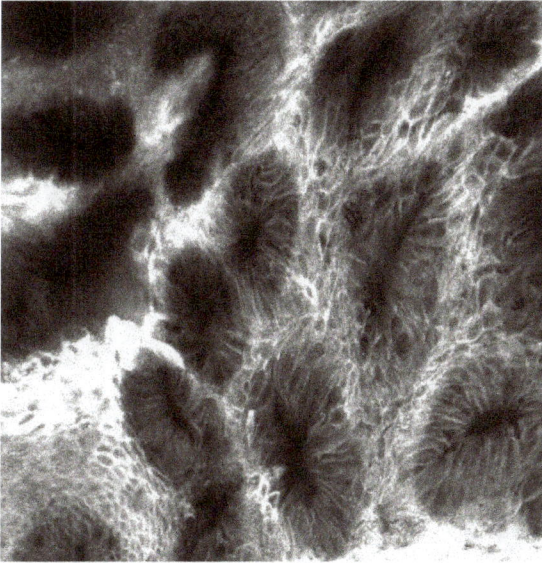

Fig. 16.4. CLE image of an adenoma showing goblet cell depletion. The epithelium of the crypts is darker with decreased mucin and goblet cells.

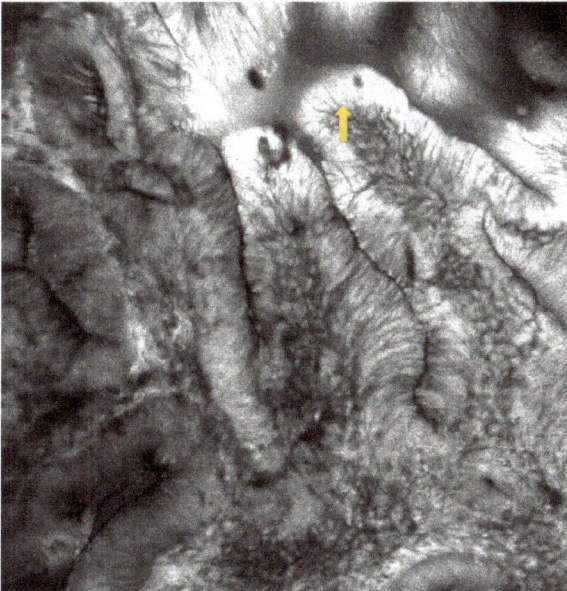

Fig. 16.5. CLE image of adenoma showing villous architecture (*arrow*).

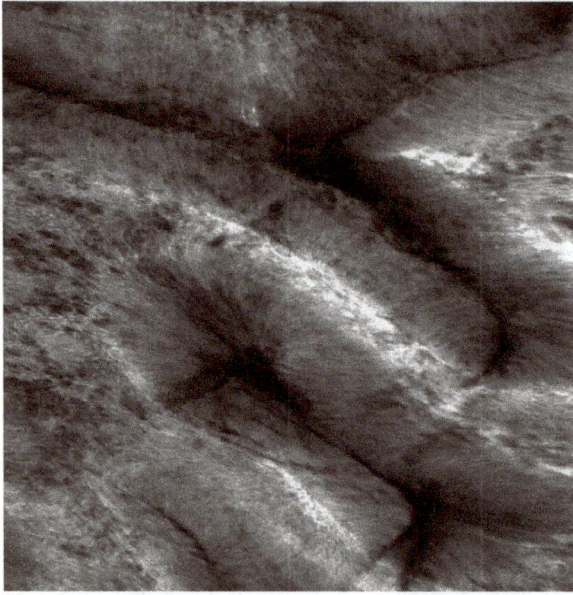

Fig. 16.6.   CLE image of adenoma showing microvascular alterations. These include dilation, increased density, and fluorescein leakage.

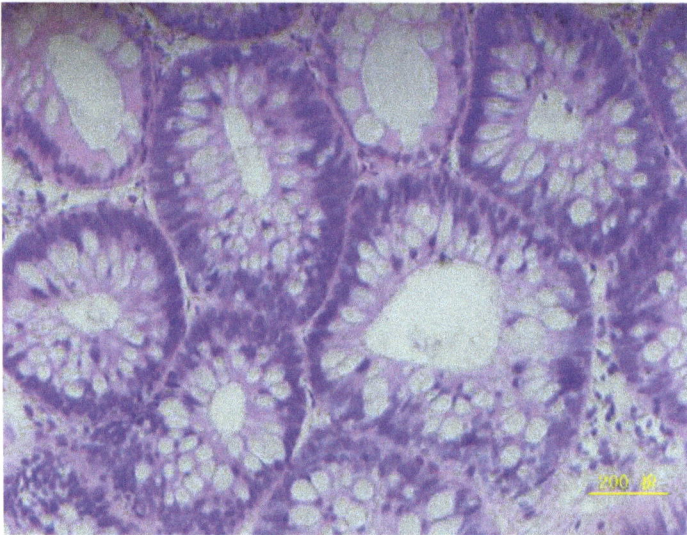

Fig. 16.7.   Histology of a hyperplastic polyp (HE × 400). The crypts are crowded with dilated openings of some crypts. Abundant goblet cells could be identified.

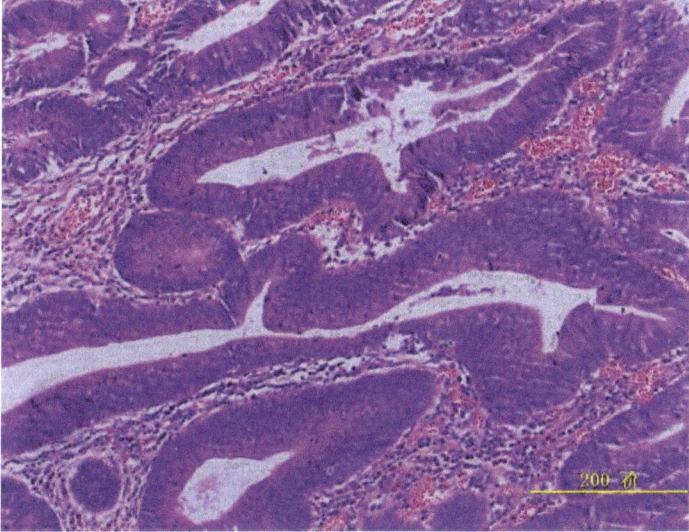

Fig. 16.8. Histology of tubular adenoma.

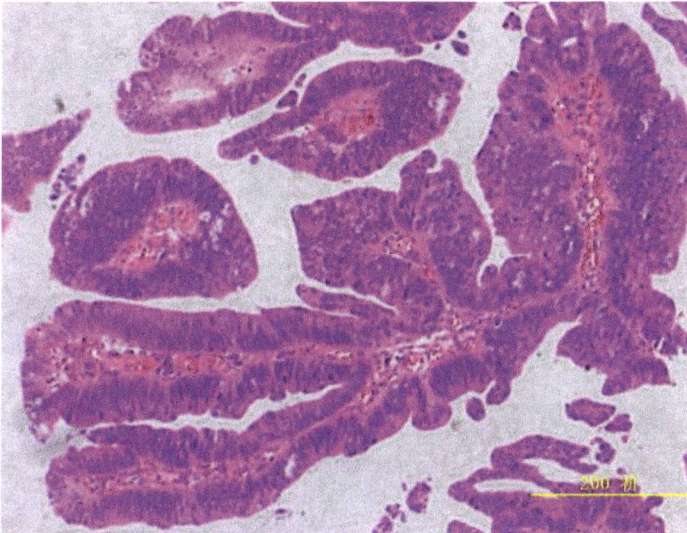

Fig. 16.9. Histology of villous adenoma (HE × 200).

References

1. Winawer S, Fletcher R, Rex D, *et al.* (2003) Colorectal cancer screening and surveillance: clinical guidelines and rationale — update based on new evidence. *Gastroenterology* **124**: 544–560.
2. Wehrmann K, Fruhmorgen P. (2000) [Removing adenomas reduces colon carcinoma risk up to 90%. Effective cancer prevention with the endoscope]. *MMW Fortschr Med* **142**: 26–29.
3. Togashi K, Konishi F, Ishizuka T, *et al.* (1999) Efficacy of magnifying endoscopy in the differential diagnosis of neoplastic and non-neoplastic polyps of the large bowel. *Dis Colon Rectum* **42**: 1602–1608.
4. Buchner AM, Shahid MW, Heckman MG, *et al.* (2010) Comparison of probe-based confocal laser endomicroscopy with virtual chromoendoscopy for classification of colon polyps. *Gastroenterology* **138**: 834–842.
5. Sanduleanu S, Driessen A, Gomez-Garcia E, *et al.* (2010) *In vivo* diagnosis and classification of colorectal neoplasia by chromoendoscopy-guided confocal laser endomicroscopy. *Clin Gastroenterol Hepatol* **8**: 371–378.

Chapter 17

Colorectal Cancer

The meaningful approaches for CLE in the diagnosis of colorectal cancer (CRC) can be summarized into four purposes: detection of inapparent cancer, reduction of biopsies, *in vivo* histology grading, and molecular diagnosis. Since detection of inapparent cancer has been discussed in the previous sections ("UC" and "CP"), this section mainly discusses the other three purposes.

Reduction of Biopsies

Colonoscopy and biopsy are standard procedures for confirming CRC, and management of CRC depends highly on findings of colonoscopy and biopsy-based histology. However, false-negative endoscopic biopsy of adenocarcinoma was reported,[1] and biopsy could influence the nonlifting sign of submucosal invasive colorectal carcinoma[2-4] and rectal carcinoids,[5] which is widely accepted as a contraindication to endoscopic mucosal resection. Although endoscopic biopsy is believed to be a safe procedure, risks of biopsy-induced epithelial misplacement in the muscularis propria[6] and metastasis[7] still exist. Our preliminary study has shown that CLE-aided biopsy could increase the sensitivity of biopsy-based histology compared to the empirical biopsy with a smaller number of biopsies per patient. However, this is only a retrospective analysis and needs to be validated in well-designed prospective studies. The value of CLE-aided biopsy is illustrated in Fig. 17.1.

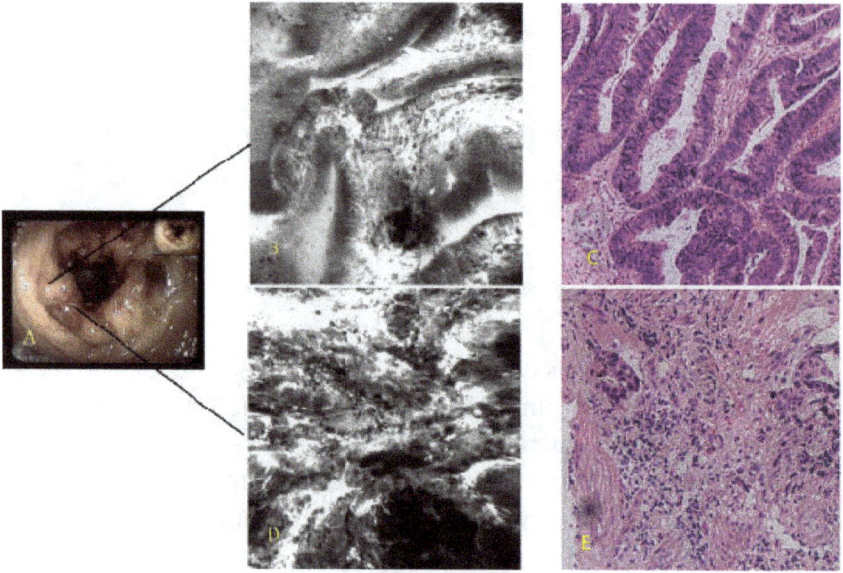

Fig. 17.1. CLE-aided biopsy for a colorectal cancer lesion. (A) White-light endoscopy image of an infiltration-type CRC lesion. (B), (C) CLE and corresponding histology based on biopsy from the outer edge of the lesion show a histology between adenoma and well-differentiated carcinoma. (D), (E) CLE and corresponding histology from the inner edge of the lesion show a histology of poorly differentiated carcinoma.

In Vivo Histology Grading

CRC is classically graded as well-differentiated carcinoma and poorly differentiated carcinoma. The two types have distinctly different pathogenesis, clinical progression, and prognosis. Under conventional endoscopy, the macroscopic types of CRC are mainly polypoid, ulceration, and infiltration types. Classically, the polypoid type is associated with well-differentiated carcinoma and the other two types with poorly differentiated carcinoma. Under CLE, the features of well-differentiated carcinoma include loss of crypts and orientation, while gland formation and the mass of epithelial cells with broken basement membrane are still visible (Fig. 17.2), and the features of poorly differentiated carcinoma include only patches of dark cells and gland formation is not visible (Fig. 17.3). The corresponding histology features of well- and poorly differentiated carcinoma are shown in Figs. 17.4 and Fig. 17.5.

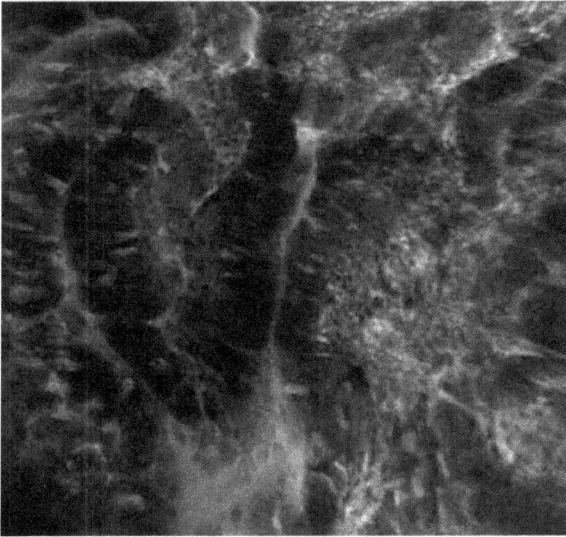

Fig. 17.2. CLE image of a well-differentiated adenocarcinoma showing the distorted but retained glands.

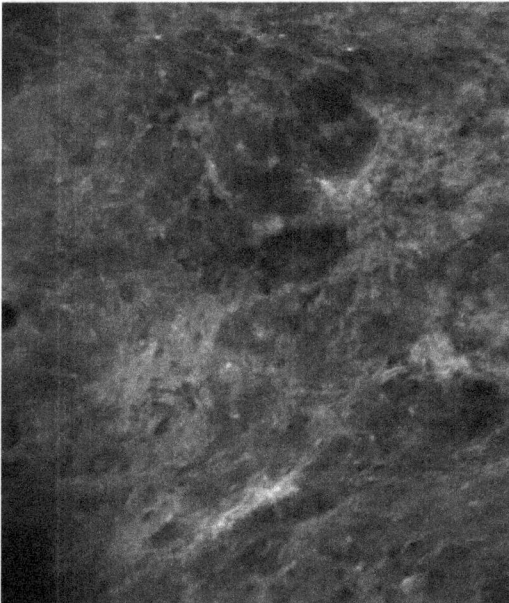

Fig. 17.3. CLE image of a poorly differentiated adenocarcinoma, showing scattered malignant cells without gland formation.

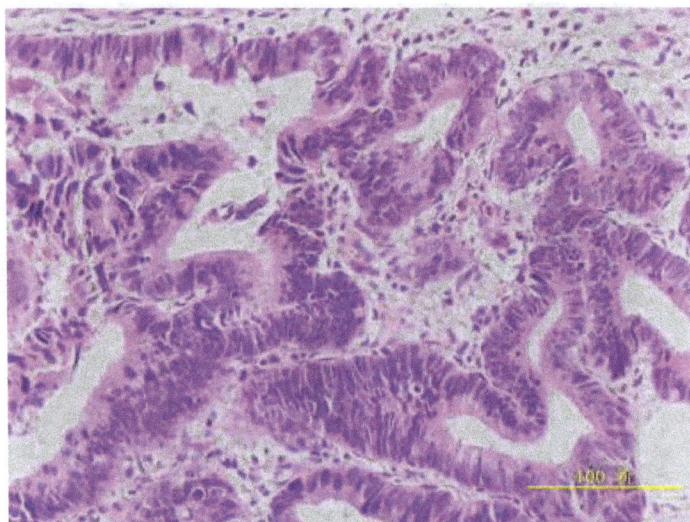

Fig. 17.4. Histology of a well-differentiated adenocarcinoma.

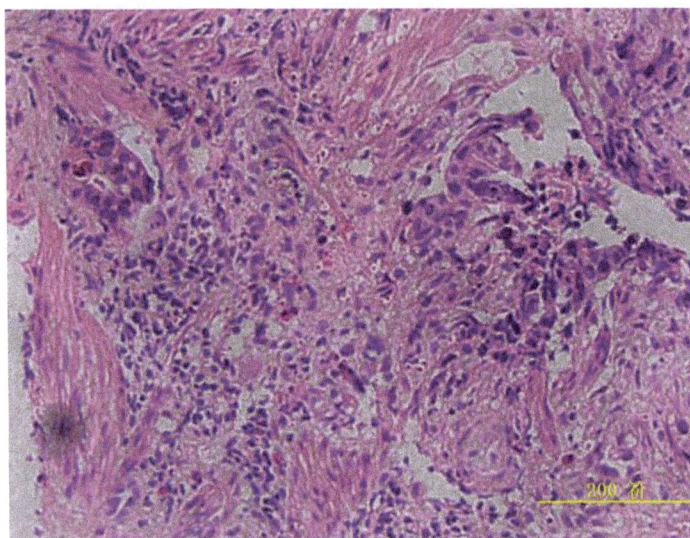

Fig. 17.5. Histology of a poorly differentiated adenocarcinoma.

Molecular Diagnosis

Molecular diagnosis for gastrointestinal tumors is not only for the purpose of confirmation diagnosis, but also for the selection of patients who will benefit from molecule-targeted treatments. The most recent study of molecular diagnosis by using CLE regarding CRC was reported by Kiesslich *et al.*[8] The targeted molecule is the epidermal growth factor receptor (EGFR), which is highly expressed in some CRC cases. Patients with EGFR-positive CRC are more likely to respond to EGFR-targeted therapies. The study showed that CLE analysis of EGFR expression in human specimens allowed distinction between neoplastic and nonneoplastic tissues.

References

1. Gillett E, Thomas S, Rodney WM. (1996) False-negative endoscopic biopsy of colonic adenocarcinoma in a young man. *J Fam Pract* **43**: 178–180.
2. Han KS, Sohn DK. (2008) Biopsy and nonlifting sign in endoscopically resectable colorectal cancers. *Gastrointest Endosc* **68**: 615.
3. Han KS, Sohn DK, Choi DH, *et al.* (2008) Prolongation of the period between biopsy and EMR can influence the nonlifting sign in endoscopically resectable colorectal cancers. *Gastrointest Endosc* **67**: 97–102.
4. Uno Y. (2008) The nonlifting sign and forceps biopsy. *Gastrointest Endosc* **68**: 1026–1027; author reply 1027–1028.
5. Cho SB, Park SY, Yoon KW, *et al.* (2009) [The effect of post-biopsy scar on the submucosal elevation for endoscopic resection of rectal carcinoids]. *Kor J Gastroenterol* **53**: 36–42.
6. Magro G, Aprile G, Vallone G, Greco P. (2007) Epithelial misplacement in the muscularis propria after biopsy of a colonic adenoma. *Virchows Arch* **450**: 603–605.
7. McCutcheon AD. (1998) Does biopsy before resection compromise prognosis in colorectal cancer? *Lancet* **352**: 910.
8. Goetz M, Ziebart A, Foersch S, *et al.* (2010) *In vivo* molecular imaging of colorectal cancer with confocal endomicroscopy by targeting epidermal growth factor receptor. *Gastroenterology* **138**: 435–446.

Part 7

FUTURE TRENDS IN CLE

Chapter 18

Current Advances and Future Trends

The development of the confocal laser endomicroscope, an imaging modality that enables *in vivo* microscopic imaging of the gastrointestinal tract, is an advance that is clearly poised to impact future endoscopic screening and diagnosis of diseases. The ultrahigh-resolution magnifying endomicroscope, with its superior optical capability to characterize mucosal and subsurface tissue at the microstructural level, has already demonstrated how it could significantly enhance the ability to detect, characterize, and diagnose many types of gastrointestinal lesions.[1] In effect, it has also heralded the advent of real-time virtual *in vivo* histopathologic diagnosis of diseases. With the confocal endomicroscope, tissue architecture, vasculature, and cellular and subcellular structures are endoscopically visualized in detail at high resolution. Studies thus far have shown that CLE detects preneoplastic and neoplastic developments in the esophagus, stomach, and colon with high degrees of accuracy. Under fluorescein-enhanced confocal imaging, intraepithelial neoplasias could be identified visually by their characteristic tubular, villous, or irregular architectures and low presence of goblet cells. Similarly, changes in inflammatory gastrointestinal disease such as ulcerative colitis, Crohn's disease and collagenous colitis could be defined by their respective confocal diagnostic characteristics.

The ability of the confocal laser endomicroscope to deliver in real time much of the diagnostic information otherwise only attainable through histopathologic examination of tissue specimens facilitates better targeting of sites for biopsy tissue acquisitions. It also offers a potentially viable alternative to excisional biopsy in cases where confirmative diagnosis could be confidently achieved *in vivo*. By helping endoscopists to make accurate diagnosis and crucial decisions on treatment options while in the process of performing the endoscopic investigations, it could expedite therapeutic interventions in diseases, thereby improving clinical outcomes. The clinical utility of this emergent imaging modality is therefore extremely promising, particularly in the endoscopic detection of early gastrointestinal cancers such as preneoplasia and neoplasia of the esophagus,[2–4] stomach,[5–7] and colorectum.[8–10]

Moving Forward and the Next Big Stride

Validation and further optimization of CLE for known applications will continue to take place. Further explorations in confocal-endomicroscopic detection of structural abnormalities in living tissue will advance fairly rapidly as investigators get more exposure to the system. Knowledge of confocal imaging features in both normal and diseased states will continue to expand, and diagnostic features for diseases will be further refined and ascertained, with the ultimate goal of attaining a universal consensus on criteria for distinguishing all the common mucosal lesions.

Studies on applications of the imaging modality in relatively uncharted territories are likely to ensue quickly too, as there remain prospects where the novel imaging system could step in to improve diagnosis or enhance understanding of disease pathogenesis. An example is the concept of epithelial gaps, which can be visualized on confocal endomicroscopy, but is not easily seen on fixed histological specimens.[11] It appears that epithelial gaps may play an important role in the pathogenesis of inflammatory bowel disease.[12] More literature on this will be available in the near future.

We may also expect some incremental technical enhancements to the current confocal imaging systems, aimed either at improving the overall functional versatility or at tailoring changes to meet specific needs. In addition to the endoscope-mounted and the probed-based confocal laser endomicroscope which are already in the market, a needle-based confocal laser endomicroscope is being evaluated.[13,14] Needle-based CLE may have utility in *in vivo* histological diagnosis of liver pathology, and may also prove to be a useful adjunct to procedures such as endoscopic ultrasound fine-needle aspiration.

There may also be novel imaging modalities which may further enhance the role of confocal endomicroscopy. Fluorescein-enhanced autofluorescence imaging has been reported to accurately differentiate between neoplastic and nonneoplastic colorectal polyps.[15] As fluorescein is the agent used for confocal endomicroscopy, there is great potential for these two modalities to complement each other.

However, the next significant stride we could make in the coming years would be in applications rather than major equipment innovation. This would most likely be the foray of CLE into the field of functional and molecular imaging — capturing on screen real-time biological phenomena at the cellular and molecular levels.

Adapting to *In Vivo* Imaging of Live Biological Processes at the Cellular and Molecular Levels

Today, with growing knowledge about the molecular biology of normal cellular functions and the changes occurring during the development of cancer and other diseases, the use of the confocal imaging modality for imaging live biological processes at both the cellular and the molecular level has great potential, not only for the early diagnosis of a disease but also for the monitoring of its development, and for its response to therapeutic treatments. Besides its high-resolution imaging capability, the confocal laser endomicroscope's adaptability to contrast-rich imaging techniques involving conjugated fluorescence probes, bioluminescent reporters, and other engineered biological tags commonly used in functional and molecular imaging would make its advancement in this area a realistic aim that is highly viable. In essence, with the envisaged implementations, it would be possible to characterize or measure in real time the physiological, cellular, and molecular processes occurring in living tissues. *In vivo* confocal imaging may be applied for two of these major purposes: (i) real-time imaging of targeted live tissues to study functional cellular processes, and (ii) imaging of targeted live tissues to identify molecular characteristics known to be related to a specific disease or stage of a disease. The former is expected to help detect early cellular changes that drive disease processes and the latter to visualize molecular changes that precede disease manifestations, usually even before structural changes become obvious under standard white-light endoscopic imaging.

Some progress has already been made in this area. *In vivo* confocal imaging of topically administered heptapeptide in patients undergoing colonoscopy showed that the fluorescein-conjugated peptide bound more strongly to dysplastic colonocytes than to adjacent normal cells.[16] In addition, confocal imaging analysis of epidermal growth factor receptor expression in human specimens accurately differentiated non-neoplasia from neoplasia.[17] These highlighted the enormous potential of CLE which could shape the future applications of this imaging technique.

Enabling Technologies, Development Accelerators and Hurdles

There is a significant potential upside for the confocal laser endomicroscope to be harnessed for functional and molecular detection and characterization of diseases. Enabling technologies are readily available. Its benchtop counterpart, the desktop confocal microscope, has long been utilized to observe cellular processes and molecular pathways in *ex vivo* biological research models. Theoretically, the same may be achieved *in vivo*, and technically, it is conceivable that the confocal endomicroscope may be functionally adapted to detect any molecule or cellular entity that can be fluorescence-tagged — from the detection of various biomarkers of diseases, to the tracking of immune and cellular functions, to the monitoring of tumor growth or regression following therapeutic interventions, and to observations of cellular apoptosis and so forth in living tissues. It must, however, be noted that technological availability and technical feasibility are not the only key to unlocking such potential. For confocal endomicroscopy to become a routine modality for clinical *in vivo* molecular imaging in human subjects, major hurdles must be surmounted. The plethora of molecular techniques and protocols currently used in benchtop studies may not be readily translated to clinical use in humans due to various constraints, primarily safety-related issues. The confocal endomicroscope is basically an epifluorescence imaging system for which the quality of the images generated relies substantially on the optimal use of contrast stains. Though, technically, the confocal endoscopic imaging system may readily adapt to the many types of exogenous probes currently applied in *ex vivo* applications, these may not all be suitable for human use. Currently, there is a paucity of non-toxic contrast media that can enhance the visual characteristics of body tissue, both normal and abnormal, and distinctly delineate neoplastic lesions from the normal surroundings. There is a dearth of properly designed clinical studies of potential agents. Brisk expansion of the confocal endomicroscope's capability, in particular the breaking of new ground in molecular diagnostic applications, will thus have to await the discovery or development of suitable highly selective contrast media. Going forward, more can then be expected in the application of the endoscopic imaging modality in advanced *in vivo* imaging, for example in the identification of specific targets such as a cancer marker or a biological process that determines the presence or stage of ongoing development of cancer or other diseases.

Looking into the Future

At the moment, the capability and potential clinical utility of the confocal laser endomicroscope are still far from being fully exploited. The future possibilities of its application to *in vivo* imaging are thus innumerable. There are shortcomings and pitfalls to be addressed, though, and evaluation of the modality's diagnostic values in large controlled, randomized clinical trials to fully assess its many promising applications is still needed. But confocal laser endomicroscopy does seem set for incorporation into routine clinical endoscopic screening, surveillance, and management of gastrointestinal diseases soon. How far and how fast it can progress in the advanced field of functional and molecular imaging will depend on how well the system can integrate with present innovations in contrast-imaging and future developments in novel approaches to image-capturing of living biological molecules.

References

1. Neumann H, Kiesslich R, Wallace MB, Neurath MF. (2010) Confocal laser endomicroscopy: technical advances and clinical applications. *Gastroenterology* **139**(2): 388–392.

2. Kiesslich R, Gossner L, Goetz M, *et al.* (2006) *In vivo* histology of Barrett's esophagus and associated neoplasia by confocal laser endomicroscopy. *Clin Gastroenterol Hepatol* **4**(8): 979–987.

3. Pohl H, Rösch T, Vieth M, *et al.* (2008) Miniprobe confocal laser microscopy for the detection of invisible neoplasia in patients with Barrett's oesophagus. *Gut* **57**(12): 1648–1653.

4. Dunbar KB, Okolo P, 3rd, Montgomery E, Canto MI. (2009) Confocal laser endomicroscopy in Barrett's esophagus and endoscopically inapparent Barrett's neoplasia: a prospective, randomized, double-blind, controlled, crossover trial. *Gastrointest Endosc* **70**(4): 645–654.

5. Guo YT, Li YQ, Yu T, *et al.* (2008) Diagnosis of gastric intestinal metaplasia with confocal laser endomicroscopy *in vivo*: a prospective study. *Endoscopy* **40**(7): 547–553.

6. Lim LG, Yeoh KG, Salto-Tellez M, *et al.* (2011) Experienced versus inexperienced confocal endoscopists in the diagnosis of gastric adenocarcinoma and intestinal metaplasia on confocal images. *Gastrointest Endosc* (in press).

7. Li WB, Zuo XL, Li CQ, *et al.* (2011) Diagnostic value of confocal laser endomicroscopy for gastric superficial cancerous lesions. *Gut* **60**(3): 299–306.

8. Kiesslich R, Burg J, Vieth M, *et al.* (2004) Confocal laser endoscopy for diagnosing intraepithelial neoplasias and colorectal cancer *in vivo*. *Gastroenterology* **127**: 706–713.

9. Buchner AM, Shahid MW, Heckman MG, *et al.* (2010) Comparison of probe-based confocal laser endomicroscopy with virtual chromoendoscopy for classification of colon polyps. *Gastroenterology* **138**(3): 834–842.

10. Xie XJ, Li CQ, Zuo XL, *et al.* (2011) Differentiation of colonic polyps by confocal laser endomicroscopy. *Endoscopy* **43**(2): 87–93.

11. Kiesslich R, Goetz M, Angus EM, *et al.* (2007) Identification of epithelial gaps in human small and large intestine by confocal endomicroscopy. *Gastroenterology* **133**(6): 1769–1778.

12. Lim LG, Neumann J, Goetz M, *et al.* (2010) Confocal endomicroscopy in the evaluation of gastric and duodenal epithelial gaps in patients with Crohn's disease and ulcerative colitis. *Gut* **59** (Suppl 3): A261.

13. Mennone A, Nathanson MH. (2011) Needle-based confocal laser endomicroscopy to assess liver histology *in vivo*. *Gastrointest Endosc* **73**(2): 338–344.

14. Becker V, Wallace MB, Fockens P, *et al.* (2010) Needle-based confocal endomicroscopy for *in vivo* histology of intra-abdominal organs: first results in a porcine model. *Gastrointest Endosc* **71**(7): 1260–1266.

15. Lim LG, Bajbouj M, von Delius S, Meining A. Fluorescein-enhanced autofluorescence imaging for accurate differentiation of neoplastic from non-neoplastic colorectal polyps: a feasibility study. *Endoscopy* (in press).

16. Hsiung PL, Hardy J, Friedland S, *et al.* (2008) Detection of colonic dysplasia *in vivo* using a targeted heptapeptide and confocal microendoscopy. *Nat Med* **14**(4): 454–458.

17. Goetz M, Ziebart A, Foersch S, *et al.* (2010) *In vivo* molecular imaging of colorectal cancer with confocal endomicroscopy by targeting epidermal growth factor receptor. *Gastroenterology* **138**(2): 435–446.

Index

www.ingramcontent.com/pod-product-compliance
Lightning Source LLC
Chambersburg PA
CBHW072257210326
41458CB00074B/2041